EASY DOES IT*
YOGA
FOR OLDER PEOPLE

ALICE CHRISTENSEN & DAVID RANKIN

"As soon as you say 'Yoga,' everybody thinks I stand on my head and do weird contortions or something. But then I show 'em this book and they say, 'Wow! We thought it was an altogether different kind of thing. . . .' And I say, 'This is something anyone can do. You don't have to be, you know, anything special. And you don't have to go anywhere to get it. You can just do it at home all by yourself.' Since I started this Yoga I feel so much more energetic, alive, and alert. And you know, it's the combination of everything in this Yoga, not just one thing, that did it—it's the whole thing. It's just grand!"

Jeanne Hrovat
an EASY DOES IT
YOGA STUDENT
age 66
Euclid, Ohio

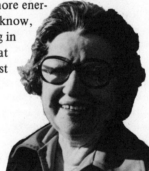

1817

Published in San Francisco by HARPER & ROW, PUBLISHERS
New York / Hagerstown / San Francisco / London
&

THE LIGHT OF YOGA SOCIETY
Cleveland / Sarasota / Paris / Srinagar

*U.S. Trademark Registration application pending for *Easy Does It*

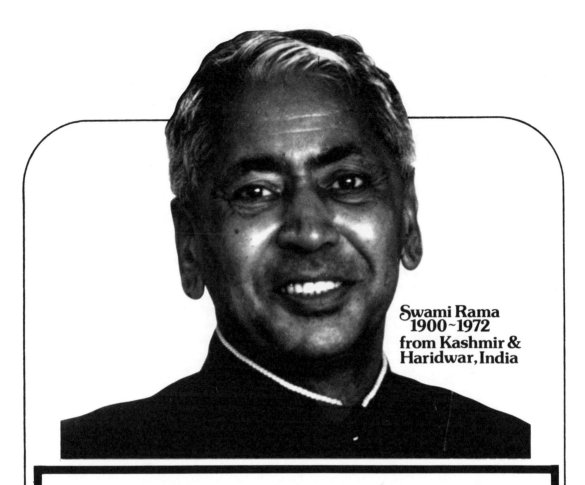

Swami Rama
1900~1972
from Kashmir &
Haridwar, India

This book is dedicated to a remarkable old man, my Guru, Swami Rama. As one of the world's greatest exponents and masters of Yoga, he embodied all the noblest traits of a truly great man: scholar, writer, poet, intellectual, musician, psychologist, philosopher, diplomat, and loving, supportive teacher. He was unassuming and humble, yet his greatness shone through all the facets of his personality like a great light in the darkness of our lives.

It is our memory of him, what he taught us, and the excellence of what he represented, that are the energy and source of this book. We have used him as the ideal example of a happy and wise older individual who is capable of inspiring and guiding younger generations. Rama did the greatest work of his life after the age of 60. He was able, through his Yoga, to take the greatest of life's sorrows and joys and make use of each for growth and wisdom. He taught and inspired us to strive for this same ability to rise above any despair and to make full use of every experience in life.

It is the light of this old man's genius, the light of Yoga, that is reflected in us and shines from the pages of this book. He was a truly great old man, who had more capacity for love, knowledge, joy, insight, and beauty than we could ever imagine.

EASY DOES IT YOGA
TABLE OF CONTENTS

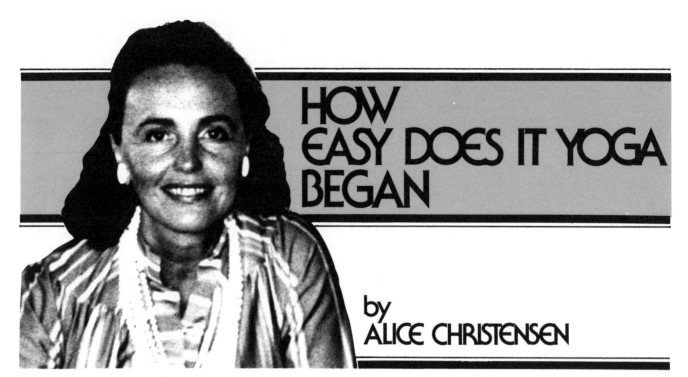

HOW EASY DOES IT YOGA BEGAN

by ALICE CHRISTENSEN

The Easy Does It Yoga program began in Cleveland, Ohio, in 1964. I had studied Yoga for many years and had just returned from seclusion in the Himalayas with my teacher Rama. In the very first Yoga class that I taught, I was shocked to find all the students were over 60 years old. One said, "We didn't tell you how old we were on the phone because we thought if you knew we were all grandparents, you wouldn't come." They, as well as most other Americans, had the mistaken idea that Yoga was exotic exercise only for young bodies. I saw for the first time in this class of brave beginners that many of the problems which robbed them of their health, vitality, and independence could be reversed. Many of their chronic health problems and negative attitudes toward themselves and growing old simply disappeared!

One class of seniors followed another, and the benefits to health, appearance, and self-esteem were obvious. A remarkable transformation was taking place. Where there had been stiff and painful bodies, there was now the spring of a more youthful step. Instead of a gray, depressed, defeated attitude, there was now joy and interest in life once again. Most importantly, my students were able to regain their self-respect and the respect of others with their mental clarity and emotional stability. My students were throwing off the rejection and fear engendered by their advancing years and were beginning to take their rightful place in society.

These observations were intensified when David Rankin and I were visiting my parents who live in a large trailer park in Florida. Living in close proximity with so many elderly people exposed us to many of the problems of both sunbelt retirees and the rural elderly of Florida's farm communities. David and I realized that these older people in Florida had the same problems as my older students in Cleveland, and that the program that I had developed in Cleveland could be tremendously effective in helping older people everywhere have happier, healthier, and more productive lives.

We published the first edition of *Easy Does It Yoga* in 1975 and began training our teachers at The Light of Yoga Society in the use of the safe techniques of Easy Does It Yoga. Demand for information about Yoga for the elderly began to increase rapidly, and the teachers of The Light of Yoga Society began giving free introductory classes in Easy

> "We didn't tell you how old we were on the phone because we thought if you knew we were all grandparents, you wouldn't come."

Does It Yoga to any interested group. In just three years, over 10,000 people attended these free classes at more than 200 locations. The culmination of all our work occurred when The Light of Yoga Society was asked to apply for a Title III grant for teaching Easy Does It Yoga throughout the Tampa Bay area on Florida's Gulf coast. A scientifically controlled study of this program's effectiveness has begun.

Easy Does It Yoga has come a long way since those first classes in 1964, and its success has demonstrated that it is a practical and effective approach to the needs of our country's elderly. Easy Does It Yoga is rapidly becoming one of the best loved self-help programs of total physical and mental fitness for older people everywhere.

AMERICA COMING OF AGE SECTION 1

Many of us fear that becoming 80 years old is worse than death itself. Researchers now feel that if we took better care of ourselves, we could live well past 100 years. However, unless we change our basic attitudes and concepts about aging, it becomes very difficult to motivate the necessary change in life style needed to live a longer, fuller, happier life. Walter Bortz, M.D., a professor at Stanford University Medical School, recently said, *"If I could convince you that to be 85 is really an exciting opportunity, and that you would be valuable to yourself and others, you would give up smoking, you would lose weight, and you would live longer. With an aggressive program of preventive medicine we would add at least ten years to the average American life span."*

In a recent survey it was shown that one third of all Americans in *every* age group considered the years between 60 and 70 as the least desirable time of their lives. Those under 65 revealed a deep prejudice against the aged. Almost universally, younger people thought the problems of the elderly were more severe than older people themselves found them to be. Ironically, the survey also revealed that the older people contributed to this negative picture of age. Even though they felt pretty good about themselves, they exaggerated the problems of poor health, loneliness, poverty, and dependency for other older people. What all this amounts to is a growing fear of age and an obsession with youth coupled with a fanatical desire to stay and look young. *"You don't look a day over 50,"* is a prized compliment, making it sound as if the days before 50 are full of beauty, while the years after 50 bring ugliness, rejection, and a growing feeling that our lives are meaningless.

IS OLD AGE WORSE THAN DEATH?

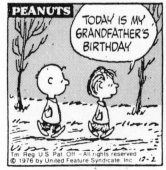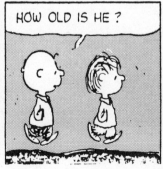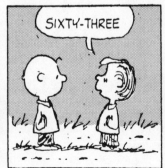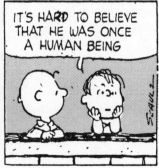

WHY DO WE HATE GROWING OLD?

Margaret Mead, the great anthropologist, felt that the high value we place on youth arose after huge waves of immigrants settled in America. Their children grew up as English-speaking citizens who were generally more successful than their foreign-born elders. The parents were less understanding of this new country and its way of life. The older generation was cut off, not only from their own families but other Americans as well. This increasing segregation prevented them from learning English, which further **...it was not an** isolated them from the **inability to work** modern cultural developments of **that segregated the** the new Amer-**elderly from the young,** ica. In **it was an incapacity** a frustrated attempt **to change.** to instill the ethnic values of their old world, they ironically began to represent the oppression and poverty from which they had fled.

The fact is that it was not an inability to work that segregated the elderly from the young; it was an incapacity to change and comprehend the new culture they were living in that drove the generations apart. In reality, the guidance of the older generation was needed as much as ever, possibly even more so. But the wisdom and insight gained during their lifetimes were increasingly ignored. This tragic process not only continues today, but worsens due to the accelerating rate of change in our society. The new technology further handicaps older Americans, obscuring the true value of their contribution to modern society.

BY THE YEAR 2000 THE OVER-60 POPULATION WILL DOUBLE.

Unless we reverse our depressing attitudes about aging, our problems will multiply dramatically. Since 1975, the number of people over 65 has increased by more than 15%. There are now 23 million Americans in this age group, and for the most part, they are not dealing with the physical and mental limitations of age or the increased stigma of our destructive national attitudes. By **People have** the year 2000, **never before been** people over 65 will **expected to live** mushroom to a staggering 31 million. This is due to a num- **this long.** ber of factors, which include the post-war baby boom as well as the fact that people in the United States are living much longer than they used to. The life expectancy in 1970

was slightly under 71 years and has since jumped to 73.2. People have never before been expected to live this long. The facts are clear: within the next fifty years we will have nearly twice as many people over 65 as we do today. If we are to avoid putting millions of Americans through unnecessary suffering, we must begin in earnest to separate the real problems from the imagined ones.

> "From what I've been able to discover elsewhere around the state of Florida and the country, *Easy Does It Yoga* is certainly a unique program for the elderly. It does things that are atypical of what you presume older people are capable of doing. It's also very successful in developing a new understanding of the whole concept of Yoga which I think has always been thought of as sort of strange. But here, we have approached the rather staid elderly community of the very conservative retiree perspective with something quite unique and avant-garde, *Easy Does It Yoga*. And it just seems to work out so beautifully. That's not only newsworthy, but also very refreshing. It's a very meaningful program for older people, and it's done very well at creating a positive image and influence. It's doing a super job!"
>
> *SCOTT WILSON, Executive Director,*
> *Tampa Bay Regional Planning Council,*
> *St. Petersburg, Florida.*

SOLVING REAL PROBLEMS

We have already discussed the fact that we picture old age as worse than it really is. We all make a big mistake in believing most older Americans waste away in nursing homes, sometimes called "feedlots for the old." The fact is that only 5% of people over 60 live in nursing homes. Over half of all older people live independently with their spouses, usually in communities where they have roots. In addition, contrary to most people's conception of the elderly as impoverished and debilitated, this description fails to describe 85% of older Americans since only 15 to 20 percent of them live below **poor health,** the poverty level.

Far more widespread and de- **retirement,** structive than these comparatively minor prob- **and inactivity.** lems are three interrelated facts of life that almost every older adult must face. These are poor health, retirement, and inactivity. These three central problems of aging feed off each other, creating a vicious cycle. Health problems often make us inactive, only making us feel worse. With poor health, retirement may become necessary, which usually contributes to inactivity and so on. We have designed the Easy Does It Yoga program to have a dramatic impact on these problems, and we think it is the most effective and unique holistic solution to these problems available today.

POOR HEALTH THE No.1 PROBLEM.

Older people today say that their number one concern is poor health. Though the elderly comprise only 10–15% of our population, the amount they spend on prescription drugs equals more than 25% of th national consumption. The medical care for our older people costs twice as much per year as for someone under 60. The last count showed this to be a frightening $1,520 per year. Three people out of four between the ages of 65 and 74 have one or more chronic illnesses. One third of all visits to physicians' offices are for chronic illnesses of the circulatory, nervous, musculoskeletal, and respiratory systems. This is significant because our students report that Easy Does It Yoga has the most effect on these areas of the body.

It is possible that the majority of health problems suffered by older people are due to unnecessary aging of important vital organs. Easy Does It Yoga teaches ways to change our life style and reactions to normal life events and reduce the strain on major systems of the body.

We all face difficulties as we go through our daily lives. Our nervous systems react to these tensions by preparing our bodies to fight or run away. In today's society we are usually unable to do either. This frustration accumulates in us and causes a tension build-up. We well know how our bodies and emotions react to such chronic tension. Our muscles and nerves become tight, and this increases anxiety, fears, and irritability. Years of tension shorten the skeletal muscles, causing poor posture, and this is responsible for the majority of back complaints. Shortened, weakened muscles are

Three people out of four between the age of 65 and 74 have one or more chronic illnesses.

the real cause for stiffness in joints, not degenerative changes in the joints themselves. Finally, tension in the muscles reduces circulation to the underlying bones and organs, resulting in the wasting of calcium in bones, cramps in muscles, poor circulation to the brain, and tension headaches. We must find new ways of dealing with the unavoidable stresses we all must face.

Easy Does It Yoga is designed to retrain the reactions to everyday situations, to rehabilitate weak, tight muscles, tendons, and ligaments, and to increase blood circulation to all parts of the body. The two areas of most noticeable improvement in our students have been relief from tension and anxiety and the ability to relax more easily. Tension reactions which speed up aging and shorten our lives are replaced with a relaxed, open-minded attitude in a stronger, healthier, more relaxed body.

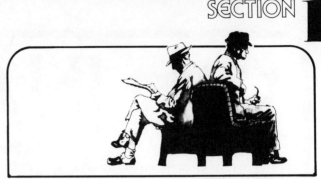

TRAUMA OF RETIREMENT

The second enormous problem we face with aging is the specter of retirement. No matter how dignified the ceremony, or how big the gold watch, choosing to retire is still seen by many of us as going out to pasture. If you are forced off the job it is doubly degrading. Our society's emphasis on production of material goods robs us of self-respect and esteem when we retire because we are viewed as worn-out machines, no longer able to produce a product. Retirement is fraught with depression, ending in suicide in extreme cases. The highest rate of suicide in the United States is among white males after they retire. These people were unable to face the transition from being a valuable part of the production system one day to the degrading status of a discarded "golden ager" the next. Much of the pain we endure when making the transition into the next stage of life could be prevented with self-help training. Reversing the idea of aging as a slow decline into

The highest rate of suicide in the United States is among white males after they retire.

oblivion would supply the necessary motivational basis for countless thousands of Americans to help themselves.

It is simply a physiological fact that our body's capacity for physical work changes as we grow older. The American obsession with material productivity leaves the older person in tremendous emotional imbalance upon retirement. How can decades of work in trades, professions, and family affairs be taken away and substituted with innocuous leisure-time activities? Are retirement and the later years of one's life meant to be filled with hollow amusements and mindless entertainment?

In contrast to this wasteful attitude toward older people, the classical Yoga traditions offer a productive, meaningful use of later years. As we get older it is essential for us to delve into the more subtle and abstract concepts of both life and death to discover what is lasting and real about ourselves. The concept of retirement in Yoga encourages a new responsibility to study the deeper issues of life. This then becomes the occupation of later years. The proper product of retirement is the growth of the individual in wisdom, insight, and leadership.■

INACTIVITY

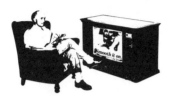

New facts about the prevention of chronic diseases have uncovered a third major problem of aging in America: a life style almost devoid of any vigorous activity. Today's older people are avoiding exercise as if it would kill them. *We now know that it is the absence of exercise that is doing the killing!*

The predominant activity of people over 55 is watching television. The A.C. Nielsen ratings estimate that the average older person watches television five hours a day. Those who not long ago worked a 40-hour week on the job or at home now spend nearly the same amount of time glued to their sets, slouched in overstuffed chairs. You might as well be bedridden! What kind of life is this for an intelligent, mature person? Just think: the commercials alone that the average older viewer will watch during the later years would be equivalent to watching Mr. Whipple squeeze the Charmin, Sarah Tucker serving Cool Whip, the heartbreak of psoriasis, and the painful itch of hemorrhoids nonstop for 1½ full years.

YOU WILL SPEND 10 OUT OF THE NEXT 20 YEARS OF YOUR LIFE EITHER SOUND ASLEEP OR WATCHING TELEVISION.

People over 55 will spend ten of their precious remaining years watching television. We're not saying that television is all bad. For many older people, television is their only window on the world. What we are saying is that the inactivity which results from watching so much television is extremely destructive. If you don't want to cut down on the amount of TV you watch, at least exercise a little bit while you're doing it. For EDY exercises you can do while watching TV commercials, see Chair Exercises, pages 33–42.

It is clear that inactivity can be directly associated with many of the problems older people usually attribute to aging. Stiffness, obesity, constipation, back pain, disc problems, weak bones, and anxiety are all related in one way or another to lack of exercise. Although high cholesterol, cigarette smoking, and high blood pressure are still regarded as primary contributors, some studies have even suggested that inactivity is an important factor in the development of the nation's number one killer, heart disease.

● **INACTIVITY IS MORE DESTRUCTIVE TO YOUR HEALTH THAN EITHER SMOKING OR OBESITY** Today everyone knows that smoking and overweight are bad for your health. But few people realize that inactivity and lack of regular exercise are more closely related to illness than smoking or obesity. Older people who are very inactive spend more weeks bedridden, visit doctors more often, have a lower opinion of their own health and live fewer years than normal. In a study of 350 obese people, only a tiny fraction (3%) of them gained weight initially from overeating. In almost 65% of the cases studied, the increase in weight was associated with inactivity due to long illness or convalescence.

IS A KILLER

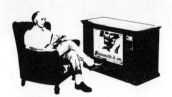

- **YOUR STIFF JOINTS MAY NOT BE DUE TO YOUR AGE** Many older people, when faced with increasingly stiff joints, blame it on their age. However, an inactive life style causes stiffness in ligaments and tendons that is indistinguishable from the changes due to age. It is, in fact, this inactivity-induced stiffness around the joints, not in the joints, which limits mobility.

- **BRITTLE BONES BREAK EASILY** Osteoporosis (porous bones) is a major health problem of the elderly, affecting 25% of the women past menopause and 10% of the men. Immobilization and prolonged bed rest can readily cause this disease of weak, porous bones. Decreased activity contributes to bones breaking for little or no apparent reason.

- **INACTIVITY CAN CAUSE TENSION, INSOMNIA, EMOTIONAL INSTABILITY, POOR APPETITE & CONSTIPATION** Muscles are designed to be used, and when not exercised, they degenerate, becoming weak, short, and tense. They accumulate energy from bodily reactions to fear, anxiety, anger, and frustration in common life situations. Exercise tends to discharge this accumulation of frustrated energy and directly affects one's emotional stability. Getting rid of tension has long been known to reduce anxiety and fears in one's emotional nature, and thus keeps us on an even emotional keel. As physical activity relaxes this nervous tension, it helps prevent insomnia, and sleep improves. Vigorous regular exercise helps one's appetite and digestion, and decreases incidence of constipation.

Older people who are very inactive spend more weeks bedridden, visit doctors more often, have a lower opinion of their health, and die younger.

- **"OH, MY ACHING BACK!"** "Oh, my aching back!" is a common refrain from older people; however, evidence from a study of 3,000 back pain cases showed that 83% of the patients had no pathological disorder. The pain was due to stiff, weak postural muscles. Tension and physical inactivity were contributing factors in many of their disabilities. In a related problem, most disease is due to poor blood supply to the spine during adult life. Inactivity is associated with this problem. Experts agree that exercise is essential for good circulation.

- **YOUR HEART IS MOSTLY MUSCLE. IT NEEDS EXERCISE TOO!** The heart and arteries consist mostly of muscle tissue. Evidence suggests that exercise helps to maintain coronary artery circulation and the flexibility of the large arteries. It is widely known that exercise improves blood circulation.

"I am in accord with your goals of activating our large numbers of older citizens who otherwise drift toward both mental and physical obsolescence. Only by maintaining a high level of dynamic physical fitness reflected in enhanced mobility, flexibility, and a renewed zest for an active life style, can our older citizens truly stay 'alive' as long as they live: alert, independent, vigorous in thought and action, with the vitality to meet each day's challenges."

LAWRENCE FRANKEL
Executive Director, Lawrence Frankel Foundation
Charleston, West Virginia

EASY DOES IT YOGA CAN HELP SAVE BILLION$

Chronic Illness

A minimum of one third of the visits to physicians by people over 60 are for the treatment of chronic conditions related to inactivity. Non-drug medical costs for older people averaged $1,400 in 1976. Sharp reductions in chronic complaints brought about by self-help procedures could possibly save as much as $250.00 per person per year. The savings for 23 million older people could be as much as $57 billion annually.

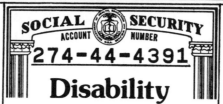

SOCIAL SECURITY
ACCOUNT NUMBER
274-44-4391

Disability

Monthly Social Security Disability payments now top $752 million due to poor health, injury, and illness. The adoption of effective self-help procedures by older people could reduce this enormous amount by 25%. This would amount to a yearly savings of $2.2 billion.

Drug Abuse

The elderly segment of our population spent about $2.8 billion on drugs in 1976. This amounts to 25% of all drug expenditures for the whole country, while the elderly comprise only 11% of the population. If increased health due to better self-care does nothing more than reduce older people's consumption of drugs to the level of the rest of our population, older people will save $1 billion of private and public money each year.

Total $avings

In a conservative estimate $9 billion could be saved annually if older people could learn such self-help procedures as Easy Does It Yoga proposes.

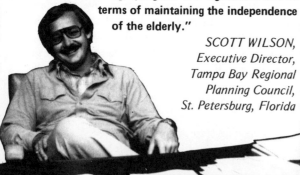

"Anything that helps older people live in their own homes and not to end up wards of the state in an institution is the goal of the Title III program of the Older Americans Act. It is more costly to society as a whole to allow older people to degenerate, if you will, to the stage where they have to be cared for in a nursing home and institutions. That's sheer economics. From a humanitarian viewpoint it is even more compelling. Any program that works in this direction should be looked at strongly, and the Easy Does It Yoga program is a significant one in terms of maintaining the independence of the elderly."

*SCOTT WILSON,
Executive Director,
Tampa Bay Regional
Planning Council,
St. Petersburg, Florida*

EASY DOES IT YOGA
CAN HELP YOU HELP YOURSELF

Although we have presented an up-to-date overview of aging in America, according to gerontological research and government statistics, as Yoga teachers we know there is no substitute for personal experience. You certainly don't need all of these numbers and aging experts to tell you how you feel. The painful realities of how you feel when you get up in the morning, and your frustration at not being able to do the things you used to be able to do are the best possible inspiration for you to do something constructive to change your life for the better. We feel that there is only one person who is responsible for your health. It isn't your pharmacist or your doctor. It is the person who looks back at you in the morning from your bathroom mirror.

How can we expect anyone else to care about the sad details of our health problems if we refuse to do anything to eliminate them? The challenge of Easy Does It Yoga is that you have the power to improve the way you feel if you have the courage and self-discipline to begin to practice.

THE EASY DOES IT YOGA PROGRAM OF TOTAL FITNESS

Easy Does It Yoga is a holistic program of daily routines consisting of exercises, breathing, relaxation, and meditation training combined with a new philosophy of aging. It is also designed to increase nutritional skills. Our goals in developing this program are to restore health and activity and to encourage a more positive view of retirement and old age. We want you to be able to live your life exactly as you would like. Through Easy Does It Yoga practices, an overall attitude of independence and growth can be maintained throughout life.

The roots of Easy Does It Yoga are grounded in classical Yoga, which is over 5,000 years old. Countless generations all over the world have benefited from these disciplines in one form or another. In ancient India, the desire of people for greater personal freedom, longer life, and heightened self-understanding gave birth to this system of physical and mental exercise. The word Yoga means to join or yoke together and it symbolizes the integration of our actions, feelings, and thoughts into one harmonious experience. Surprisingly, the ideal age to begin to practice Yoga was said to be 53, the age in India which marks the passage into a new stage of life, that of contemplation and self-discovery. In view of the fact that Yoga was traditionally practiced by older people, and since it was designed to develop better physical and mental health, it seems to be a perfect tool to use in correcting our modern problems of poor health, retirement, and inactivity.

THE 5 MAJOR ASPECTS OF EASY DOES IT YOGA

The Easy Does It Yoga program achieves a condition of total fitness through training in five different areas. Each aspect of EDY training engages different parts of your body and mind.

1. EXERCISES Gentle stretching, strengthening, and balancing.

2. BREATHING Slow and deep breathing exercise to improve the respiratory system.

3. RELAXATION & MEDITATION Step-by-step procedures to release tension throughout the body and improve concentration. Training in stillness of the body, emotions, and mind to develop a bright, fresh outlook.

4. PHILOSOPHY Yogic concepts of age to help you optimize your later years.

5. NUTRITION Low-budget ways to boost your health by improving traditional diets.

1. EDY EXERCISE

"In my observations, *Easy Does It Yoga* is a very positive activity for older people to be involved in. Most older people don't get very much exercise, yet they really approach *Easy Does It Yoga* with enthusiasm. In my opinion, anything that enhances the physical and mental well-being of older people enhances their whole life style. The approach of *Easy Does It Yoga* is very positive, and the benefits become obvious within a relatively short period of time."

Maeve Foster, Executive Director, Area Agency on Aging, Council for Human Services of South Central Florida, Ft. Myers, Florida

The first component of the Easy Does It Yoga program is exercise. We have modified traditional Yoga exercises into a safe, gentle, and gradual system which does not require great limberness or stamina. These exercises consist of a short series of bends, lifts, and twists performed with specific breathing patterns. These can be done while standing, seated in a chair, on a bed, in a bathtub, watching television, or even in a wheelchair. We have carefully tailored the exercises so that they can be done by anyone regardless of physical limitations. This has allowed blind, disabled, and even severely handicapped older students to benefit from regular exercise which many of them thought they could no longer do. All of these exercises are designed to work around the common limitations of age.

Do not allow yourself to think that you are too old, stiff, or disabled to begin exercising again. In fact, many studies and our own personal experience have undeniably proven that the participants who have been the least active and who are the most damaged by inactivity are the ones who have benefited the most from an exercise program. It may be the lack of exercise in your life that is responsible for much of your pain, stiffness, tension, obesity, insomnia, anxiety, and depression. Remember that the amount of exercise you get every day is the single most important factor in maintaining your good health.

The primary aspect of any exercise program is that it be enjoyable—otherwise you

You are not too old, too stiff or disabled to begin exercising again.

will not continue doing it. We are well aware of the fact that most of us loathe exercise, but you will love doing Easy Does It Yoga exercises. After doing your exercise program each day, you should not be tired out at all, but instead feel refreshed and energized. In short, these exercises are for everyone. They can be enjoyed by the active older person who loves to jog or play vigorous sports as well as by people who may be greatly overweight or who have never done any sort of regular physical exercise or activity. Our students give the best testimony to the fact that they enjoy Easy Does It Yoga, because on the average they practice their exercises ten minutes longer every day than we suggest!

OBJECTIVES OF EDY EXERCISES

1. MOBILITY Loosen stiff, frozen joints and strengthen and limber the muscles, tendons, and ligaments.

2. IMPROVED FUNCTIONING OF THE CIRCULATORY SYSTEM Increase blood supply to head, arms, and legs, normalize blood pressure, and ease the strain on the heart.

3. BETTER BREATHING Strengthen muscles of respiration, loosen the chest wall, and restore elasticity of lung tissue.

4. IMPROVED FUNCTIONING OF DIGESTIVE AND GENITAL-URINARY SYSTEMS Stimulate smooth muscle tone of digestive and eliminative organs by deep internal massage to help constipation, bladder and prostate problems, and improve sex life.

5. INCREASED ACTIVITY Restores confidence to enable re-entry into an energetic, satisfying life style.

6. WEIGHT CONTROL Relieve depression and anxiety that trigger overeating, and strengthen willpower to eat only the calories needed to maintain correct weight.

7. BETTER COORDINATION Restore "kinesthetic awareness" (body sensitivity), improved balance, and better integration of the nerves which control body movement.

8. REDUCED ANXIETY Reduction of fear and nervousness by released tensions and frustrations that build up in the body.

2. EDY BREATHING EXERCISES

The Easy Does It Yoga exercises for the respiratory system are the most unique aspect of the entire program. Many older people only breathe with the upper third of their lungs, and these breathing exercises retrain your body to use the lungs to their fullest capacity. Many of our students tell us that the breathing exercises are their favorite part of the course, and they do them while watching television, walking, bathing, or even lying in bed.

Better breathing can add years to your life. Breath is vital for life, yet we give it much less consideration than food, water, and shelter. We usually take it completely for granted unless something like asthma, emphysema, bronchitis, or pneumonia develops, and then we value each and every breath. You need an incredible 2,300 gallons of air to breathe every day. If you are without breath for only a

few minutes the brain cells begin to perish, and death results unless breath starts again soon.

When you were 30, statistics say you probably breathed 135 gallons of air each hour, and if you are over 65, you are now breathing just 95 gallons of air. Your daily breathing now supplies you with nearly 1,000 gallons less air per day! We can regain a great deal of that lost 40 gallons of air per hour by strengthening the muscles in the back and chest, by loosening up the chest wall with special exercises for the body and by controlled breathing exercises. Isn't it possible that some aging problems that we take for granted, such as confusion, fatigue, and depression, are due only to poor breathing?

As we age we tend to breathe more with the

upper lung area and ignore the lower. Unfortunately, the blood circulation which picks up the oxygen accumulates more in the lower lung. It's as if we have all the air upstairs while all the blood is downstairs. As a result, the blood's content of oxygen tends to decrease with age, an important factor in the development of confused, muddled thinking, a symptom of senility. Lung efficiency normally decreases further when lying down and nighttime confusion frequently results from decreased oxygen levels during sleep. The brain requires three times as much oxygen as the rest of the body, so it is affected the most by lower blood levels. The sluggish, depressed moods of many of our older students disappear when they begin to breathe better.

The retraining of the muscles in the diaphragm and the abdomen brings each breath lower into the lungs where more of the blood circulates. You will learn to breathe easier, deeper and slower, getting more of the fresh energy of life to the brain and body. You will feel better about your life because your mind will be brighter and more alert. Don't five or ten minutes of breathing exercises seem like a small price to pay for the chance to add healthy, happy years to your life? Give it a try!

OBJECTIVES OF EDY BREATHING EXERCISES

1. **STRENGTH** Increase the strength of all the muscles and nerves used in breathing.
2. **GREATER LIMBERNESS** Increase the flexibility of the joints where the ribs join the breastbone in the front, and the spine in the back.
3. **GREATER VITAL CAPACITY** Increase the volume of air that one can breathe.
4. **INCREASED DAILY BREATH VOLUME** Increase the amount of air breathed every day.
5. **RAISE OXYGEN & ENERGY LEVEL** Increase the amount of available oxygen to all parts of the body, raising one's energy levels.
6. **BREATHE EASIER** Lower the respiration rate by deepening the air flow into the total lung space and purify the lung tissues.
7. **REDUCE HEART STRAIN** Decreasing the number of breaths per minute and increasing oxygen supply reduces the effort and strain on the heart.

3. EDY RELAXATION & MEDITATION

Relaxation is a valuable tool to eliminate the accumulated frustration and strain present in everyday activities. Easy Does It Yoga teaches you a process of mentally visualizing the different parts of the body to locate tension spots and gently relax them. This is taught in a variety of body positions so it is more applicable to normal life activities. Students learn to relax while standing, sitting, and lying down, and they are encouraged to practice the technique at various times during their day. After relaxing the body, the meditation training takes over to relax and quiet the mind. The effect is to produce a state of deep silence and peace which is intensely pleasurable. Both of these practices improve concentration skills to help memory and to make daily life more efficient.

OBJECTIVES OF EDY RELAXATION & MEDITATION

1. **LESS TENSION & STRESS** Learn how to quiet the mind and relax tension in the body without medicine.
2. **IMPROVE CONCENTRATION & AWARENESS**
3. **INCREASED COPING SKILLS** Develop more effective stress coping skills and approaches.
4. **REDUCE ANXIETY, IRRITABILITY & NERVOUSNESS**
5. **DEVELOP A POSITIVE SELF-IMAGE**

4. EDY PHILOSOPHY

Yoga is not based on any original book or scripture; instead, its ideas were handed down orally from teacher to student for thousands of years. Although the earliest written record probably did not appear until 600 B.C., Yoga predates all the philosophies of the world. The goal of this philosophy is self-understanding and the growth of a harmoniously balanced individual. This system, then, is more than just a collection of ideas – the very essence of Yoga philosophy is experience.

The ideas and growth associated with Yoga have tremendous value for older Americans. As you begin to know yourself better, your self-esteem and leadership ability emerge. You will ultimately discover something at the very core of your being which does not change, or grow old. In Yoga this is called the Self, and it is the real support of the individual. As Self-awareness grows, you become more resistant to the negative attitudes of depression, fear, and despair associated with growing old and begin to find deep beauty and solace inside yourself.

OBJECTIVES OF EDY PHILOSOPHY

1. **INCREASE SELF-RESPECT & POSITIVE SELF-IMAGE** while becoming more tolerant of others.
2. **ENHANCE MATURITY** Develop more mature concepts of life and death.
3. **DIMINISH FEARS** Develop greater freedom from incapacitating fears, and explore your full potential.

5.EDY NUTRITION

Recent research has illustrated marked deficiencies and imbalances in the diets of many older people. It is very clear that the American high-sugar, high-fat, low-fiber diet is prematurely killing us. In an article for the medical journal *Geriatrics,* John T. Kelly, M.D., states, "Overconsumption of . . . saturated fats . . . cholesterol, sugar, salt and alcohol has been related to six of the ten leading causes of death. They are heart disease, cancer, cerebrovascular disease, diabetes, arteriosclerosis, and cirrhosis of the liver." Low-income people, particularly those over 65, may be especially attracted to high-fat, high-sugar diets. It is estimated that at least 20% of all adults in the U.S. are overweight to a degree that may impair health and longevity.

The Easy Does It Yoga program presents an attractive alternative to our unhealthy American diet based on the use of more traditional foods and simple ways of preparing them. Far from being a new "health food" diet, these suggestions resemble the way we ate before food technology became such a big business. We have designed a flexible diet substantially lower in all fat and higher in unrefined carbohydrates. Refined sugar foods are limited as well as the use of canned and frozen foods which are expensive and lower in vitamins and fiber than fresh fruits and vegetables. Such a diet is healthier, cheaper and lower in calories. It is our intention to eliminate the common diseases of malnutrition affecting millions of older people. Conditions such as obesity, osteoporosis, diabetes, arthritis, cardiovascular disease, anemia, constipation and many nonspecific complaints such as confusion, poor appetite, melancholy and listlessness can be helped by an improvement in the diet, following the Easy Does It Yoga guidelines.

OBJECTIVES OF EDY NUTRITION

1. **HOW TO** recognize and purchase nutritious foods on a limited income.
2. **HOW TO** store and prepare foods for best nutrition.
3. **HOW TO** recognize the most common nutritional diseases and what to do about them.

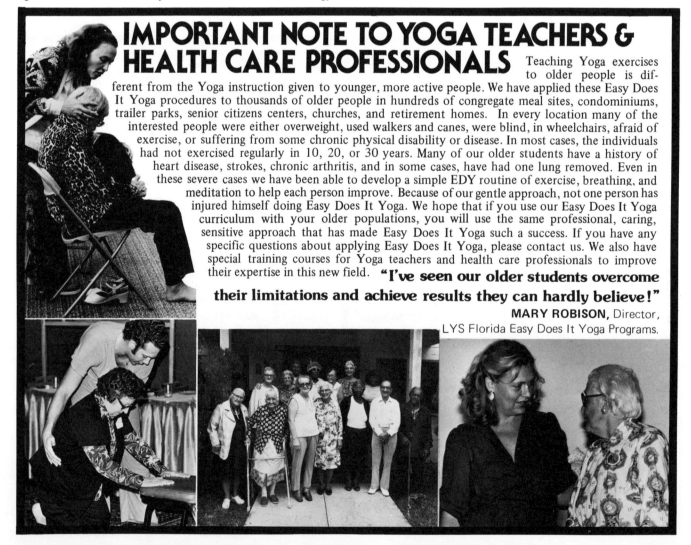

IMPORTANT NOTE TO YOGA TEACHERS & HEALTH CARE PROFESSIONALS
Teaching Yoga exercises to older people is different from the Yoga instruction given to younger, more active people. We have applied these Easy Does It Yoga procedures to thousands of older people in hundreds of congregate meal sites, condominiums, trailer parks, senior citizens centers, churches, and retirement homes. In every location many of the interested people were either overweight, used walkers and canes, were blind, in wheelchairs, afraid of exercise, or suffering from some chronic physical disability or disease. In most cases, the individuals had not exercised regularly in 10, 20, or 30 years. Many of our older students have a history of heart disease, strokes, chronic arthritis, and in some cases, have had one lung removed. Even in these severe cases we have been able to develop a simple EDY routine of exercise, breathing, and meditation to help each person improve. Because of our gentle approach, not one person has injured himself doing Easy Does It Yoga. We hope that if you use our Easy Does It Yoga curriculum with your older populations, you will use the same professional, caring, sensitive approach that has made Easy Does It Yoga such a success. If you have any specific questions about applying Easy Does It Yoga, please contact us. We also have special training courses for Yoga teachers and health care professionals to improve their expertise in this new field. **"I've seen our older students overcome their limitations and achieve results they can hardly believe!"**
MARY ROBISON, Director, LYS Florida Easy Does It Yoga Programs.

We have always realized a need for hard facts about what actually happens to older people as a result of daily Yoga practice. The greatest resistance and negativity we faced in applying our program was not from older people themselves, but from administrators and aging specialists responsible for some of their activities. These people, however, were soon won over by the enthusiasm of the older students. We realize that enthusiasm is not enough. We need to establish a concrete data base to clearly demonstrate exactly what happens as people start to practice Yoga.

We received expert help in setting up a program of fact gathering. Durand Jacobs, Ph.D., a well-known psychologist, offered assistance because of his deep belief in the importance of self-help procedures. We used questionnaires which measure broad changes in the body, emotions, and mind, and administered them before the Yoga training. We retested our students at intervals as they continued to practice. After beginning our Title III Easy Does It Yoga program in Florida,

A PRELIMINARY EVALUATION OF EASY DOES IT YOGA

David Haber, Ph.D., a professor at the University of South Florida, helped us simplify other health questionnaires so they would be more usable in Florida's rural communities. We are very grateful for the help of these two fine scientists.

We have involved more than 300 of our older students in our preliminary research. The average age of this group is 71 years, and they had about nine years of formal education. 80% of the students were female. Four in ten were married, and the rest were single, widowed, or divorced. At the beginning of the course these people were primarily interested in becoming more "limber, strong, and healthy," in "learning to relax," and in "improving their concentration." After only five to eleven weeks of practice, they saw a significant improvement in these areas.

Our students felt that Easy Does It Yoga was extremely pleasant to do and gave them relief from a whole range of problems. We feel that this is the most significant criterion for the evaluation of any self-help program.

REPORTS OF GREATER LIMBERNESS, STRENGTH, & HEALTH

The important benefits our students have noticed can be grouped into four categories:

1. **Musculoskeletal System** Pain in the back, arms and legs, as well as cramps, are usually due to weak and tense muscles and poor circulation. Our students found that their complaints of such problems reduced markedly and that there was an overall reduction in pain caused by muscle tension.

2. **Respiratory System** They also noticed improved functioning of the nose and throat, as they were less bothered by running and bleeding noses or constant coughing.

3. **Nervous System** Many students experienced fewer problems of numbness and tingling in the arms and legs. They also had fewer severe headaches, reduced dizziness, and less twitching in the face, head, and shoulder area.

4. **Emotions** Emotionally there were large reductions in anxiety symptoms such as nervousness, being easily irritated, and doing things on impulse. Muscle tensions were relieved, making anxiety less of a problem. Our older students reported getting along better with other people, as they felt less need to be on guard with their friends and felt less critical of them. Self-esteem increased as feelings of uselessness and being "no good" diminished. Many of our older students have also reported a renewed interest in sex.

WHAT DOES ALL THIS MEAN ?

Until the controlled studies now underway are completed, the evaluation lacks comparison with changes which normally occur in older people. These controlled studies are underway, involving the participants in our Title III program on the Gulf coast of Florida. We realize that this preliminary evaluation cannot be considered conclusive, but we do have some definite results that are very promising.

1. There are consistent reports of **reduced anxiety symptoms**, particularly those which stem from tension in muscles and nerves.

2. Our students consistently report **reduced pain and stiffness in the back, legs, neck, and shoulders.**

3. Most encouraging are reports that after practicing Easy Does It Yoga they are **less bothered by irritability, anger, and intolerance,** and as a result, are able to **get along better with other people and enjoy their company more.**

4. Our older students had **more self-respect and felt more confident in dealing with the problems of their lives.**

5. Our older students tell us that they actually do their Easy Does It Yoga practices two or three times as long as we suggest in the program. **This indicates that Easy Does It Yoga is not boring and is fulfilling a need.**

"More than enthusiastic testimonials must be offered to convince health professionals and administrators that simple Yoga exercises can reduce somatic and psychological complaints. What impressed me most on first meeting the Directors of The Light of Yoga Society was their willingness for an objective evaluation by an unbiased third party and their agreement to my condition that all findings be released for publication whatever the outcome. The findings from the research program, which I subsequently designed, have tended to support their initial observations. This kind of research is an essential prerequisite for identifying and refining reliable methods for training both young and old in low-risk and high-gain self-help procedures."

Durand F. Jacobs, Ph.D., Diplomate in Clinical Psychology, Prof. of Psychology, Loma Linda University, Loma Linda, California

EFFECTS & BENEFITS SECTION 2

"The response to Easy Does It Yoga at the Site Centers has been overwhelming both in terms of the large numbers of older people wanting to participate and the results they receive from the practice—super results. I have actually observed them practicing in the classes and have, in several cases, seen the changes occur in the older students. It's been of particular interest to me to see how involved these people get in Easy Does It Yoga. They aren't forced to do their Yoga every day, and yet they want to. So they do it regularly. That's a big change in the attitudes of older people. We look forward to next year when we can expand the Easy Does It program."

GRACE GANLEY, Chief, Division on Aging,
Tampa Bay Regional Planning Council, Tampa, Florida.

We are firmly convinced of the practical benefits that Yoga offers people of all ages, and we lecture, instruct, and counsel Yoga students all over the world. One of the most satisfying and astounding facets of our work has been observing the positive changes that occur in our older students. In many instances, the physical limitations of the individuals have been so great that the first step was to simply convince them to try a little. In fact, in even the most severe cases, a few simple exercises that the person could do in a chair or bed were enough to encourage them to do them again throughout the day. Then they would do them a little bit more, until finally they realized they could do Yoga easily and were greatly encouraged.

The benefits in some cases are so astounding that only by meeting the individuals and hearing in their own words what their Yoga means to them, can you get a realistic picture of Easy Does It Yoga. In this section and throughout the book we have included some candid interviews with some of our EDY students so that you may get to know them as we have. If you are concerned about your own health and well-being, or perhaps that of a loved one, this section may prove helpful and give you courage to try this simple formula for health and fitness. Each page centers around a specific area of complaints common to many older people. At the bottom of each page you will find suggestions of specific Yoga exercises and procedures that may prove beneficial to you.

**ALICE CHRISTENSEN &
DAVID RANKIN
designers of EASY DOES IT YOGA**

photo: Venice Gondolier

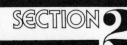
"I USED TO HAVE TO ROCK BACK AND FORTH 5 OR 6 TIMES TO GET OUT OF THIS CHAIR. NOW I CAN GET RIGHT UP."

EMMA MAE MAYS / 63 / PALMETTO, FLORIDA

photos by Evelyn England

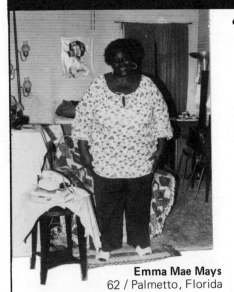

Emma Mae Mays
62 / Palmetto, Florida

"I was in such bad shape that all I'd feel like doing was get out of bed and sit in this chair. I'd put on my duster and keep it on all day. I couldn't even get dressed. I'd just sit and watch TV, wouldn't even put a comb to my head. Then when the sun went down, I'd go back to bed. Now since this Easy Does It Yoga I get up and jump in my car and go everywhere. I go all over the place again, driving my neighbors everywhere. **I'm involved in this community again!**"

"It's helped me in particular to be able to sweep the floor better. I lost my sight two years ago and what with my stiffness and all, I didn't very often sweep or vacuum the floor before I started this Yoga exercise. Now I can get right down to plug in the vacuum and then I can get right back up. Isn't that something?"

Ada Duffy
77
Plant City, Florida

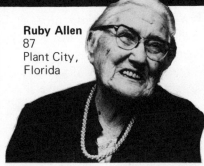

Ruby Allen
87
Plant City,
Florida

"Used to be I could only walk one way to the store, two blocks away; coming back I felt about dead. I'd have to stop and have someone come get me. Now I can go all the way to the grocery store and back because those Yoga exercises have brought new strength into my legs. I can even stand up all the way through singing two hymns in church again!"

"I was terribly short of breath— sometimes I couldn't walk much because of that. Now that I do that long breath, well, it helps, because **I'm getting around a little better!**"

What you should do.

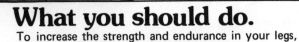

To increase the strength and endurance in your legs, do these exercises every day:

Also remember to do your knee, ankle, and lower back massage on pages 75 and 76.

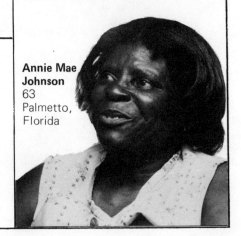

**Annie Mae
Johnson**
63
Palmetto,
Florida

• BREATHING BETTER •

"BELIEVE ME, WHEN YOU FEEL THAT EACH BREATH MAY BE YOUR LAST... THAT'S STRESSFUL!"

DOROTHY WILD / 69 / SARASOTA, FLORIDA

"Well I have bronchitis and asthma, and I also have emphysema. which makes it hard to breathe, especially if you get an infection. I can't just give in to these physical limitations like some folks do just give up— then things really get worse. If I don't feel like I'm doing something about it I get depressed and stressful. And believe me, when you feel that each breath may be your last, that's stressful! The two best things are the Yoga postures, to facilitate the removal of fluid from the lungs, and the strengthening of the breathing muscles. I have to work hard at breathing. I get short of breath quickly. I even have trouble doing light housework like vacuuming or sweeping floors because sometimes it makes me so short of breath that I have to lie down. **My Yoga does and has definitely helped me increase my breath capacity.**"

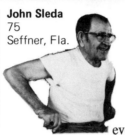

John Sleda
75
Seffner, Fla.

"I do the breathing exercises quite a bit, sometimes even in church. Both my wife's and **my breathing has improved a lot.**"

Jim Chesser / 77
Dover, Florida

"Oh, yeah. That breathing's helped. Helps you breathe easier and your breath's not so short."

"I would just lie in bed at night and my breath just seemed so shallow that it made it difficult to fall asleep. **It wasn't until I started this Yoga that I ever learned how to breathe deeply?**"

Josephine Vidmar / 70
Cleveland, Ohio

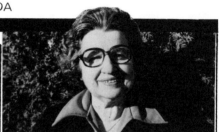

Jeanne Hrovat / 66 / Euclid, Ohio

"It's made me more alert. It seems like I get more air, more energy, and oh, I used to get so tense. Sometimes I get really angry, especially if I'm around people who are very trying. My breathing has helped me tolerate them a lot better. I can be more patient with them. **Now, when I get angry, I just take a few deep, slow breaths,** and do you know, that's what helps me tolerate them. I come out of that angry feeling and just relax. My whole tone changes, and I can talk to them real close, just real gentle. Before, I'd like to have screamed at them and told them off. I can just handle situations like that better now because of my breathing. Isn't that odd?"

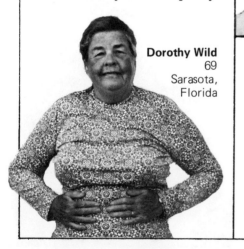

Dorothy Wild
69
Sarasota,
Florida

What you should do.

To improve your breathing, go straight to **Section 7, Breathing Exercises,** on pages 79–86. You also need to do exercises which limber and strengthen the chest, like the **Seated Twist, page 40,** and the **Easy Bridge, page 54.**

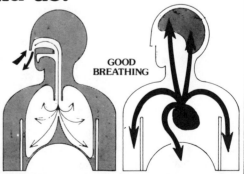

GOOD BREATHING

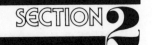
• ARTHRITIS & STIFF JOINTS •

"I'D HAVE TO HOLD ONTO THE BANISTER AND GO DOWNSTAIRS LIKE A LITTLE BABY DOES. I FELT SO DOPEY..."

JEANNE HROVAT / 66 / EUCLID, OHIO

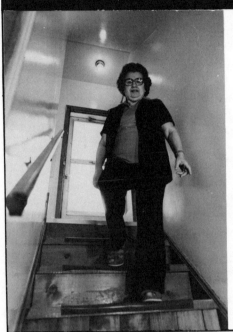

"My knees used to be so arthritic; you may not know what the pain's like, but I'm telling you, I used to have to hold onto the banister and just go down stairs like a little baby. I had to put both feet on the step, hold on, and then slowly go to the next stair. I felt so dopey. **Now I can go up and down the stairs almost normal like.** It still hurts a little bit, you know, but I can go down without holding on. Isn't that marvelous?"

Jeanne Hrovat
66 / Euclid, Ohio

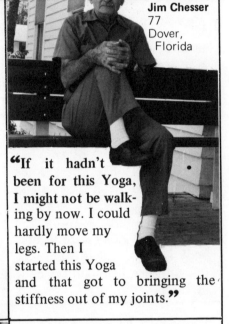

Jim Chesser
77
Dover,
Florida

"If it hadn't been for this Yoga, I might not be walking by now. I could hardly move my legs. Then I started this Yoga and that got to bringing the stiffness out of my joints."

"I suffer from arthritis. Not so much in my joints like some folks, mine's in the thick part of my thigh. At night it aches just like a toothache. **I know it's my Yoga that's made the difference** because I'd go to the doctor and get shots and medicine, but it didn't go away. Since my Yoga, it doesn't seem to bother me as much."

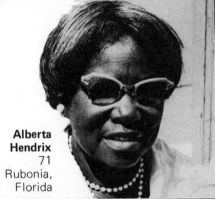

Alberta Hendrix
71
Rubonia,
Florida

"When I started this I couldn't bend this leg and knee—had arthritis and rheumatism in it for about 18 years. **This Yoga sure helped.** It's really better."

Ada Duffy
77
Plant City,
Florida

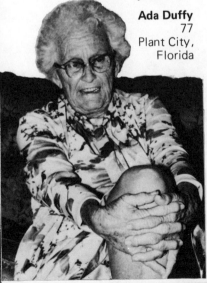

What you should do.

These exercises are excellent for reducing pain in the joints:

KNEE SQUEEZES—p. 44, 53, 68;
SHOULDER SHRUGS—p. 33;
HEAD ROTATIONS—p. 36
ARM REACHES/ROTATIONS—p. 37/38;
STANDING REACHES—p. 43/FOOT FLAP—p. 52.

You should also remember to do the **tub poses on page 77,** and all of the **massage procedures on pages 75—76.** There are also some **diet tips for arthritis sufferers on page 103.**

• CONSTIPATION & INDIGESTION •

"I'M NOT CONSTIPATED ANYMORE NOW THAT I DO MY YOGA EXERCISES."

METTIE BRANNON / 67 / PLANT CITY, FLORIDA

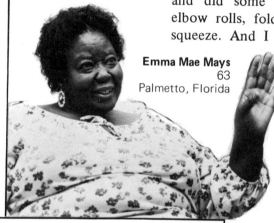

Mettie Brannon
67
Plant City,
Florida

"I had a terrible problem. I had a real time with constipation for years. I'm not constipated anymore now that I do the knee squeezes and my other Yoga exercises. I like that knee squeeze. I do it in the bed and on the side of the bed, on a chair —just anywhere—**even on the commode. I don't care if anybody knows it!** This is the best thing for me. I wouldn't trade it for anything!"

"I had a gas pocket here on my left side giving me terrible pain which lasted for three days. I even went to the emergency room at the hospital one night it was so bad, but they didn't help me get relief. I was in such misery with the pain. Then I remembered and did some of my Yoga exercises— elbow rolls, folded pose, and that knee squeeze. And I declare, if I didn't start feeling so much better right then! I just couldn't believe it. **Now I hardly ever get that gas, and I used to have it all the time.** If it acts like it's coming back, I just get in my bed and do those knee squeezes."

Emma Mae Mays
63
Palmetto, Florida

"I had to take something all the time for constipation. Yeah, every other day I'd take those little chocolate whatchacallits. They'd help for a while, but then it'd come right back. But this drawing up the knees and squeezing and things like that's done good for me. **I haven't had to take anything in seven months.** Sure has saved my husband some drugstore money. Not only that, but I love cheese, and now I can eat cheese again!"

Annie Mae Johnson / 63 / Palmetto, Florida

"Every morning I'd have terrible indigestion. And you know what's helped? Now I do those arm reaches with my fists up towards the ceiling and **that gets rid of it right away!"**

Katrina Price
68
Plant City,
Florida

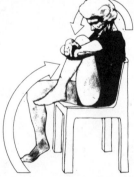

What you should do.

The best exercises for improved digestion and to relieve constipation are:

ELBOW TO KNEE	p. 39	SEATED FULL BEND BREATH	p. 42
SHOULDER TO KNEE	p. 39	SEATED FULL BEND TWIST	p. 42
KNEE SQUEEZE	p. 53	SEATED TWIST	p. 40
SEATED KNEE SQ.	p. 41	FOLDED POSE	p. 38

You also need to make some **simple changes in your diet by following the suggestions on pages 105 and 106.**

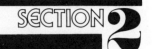
"AFTER ABOUT SIX WEEKS OF PRACTICE MY BLOOD PRESSURE HAD DROPPED TO 124/80."

DORIS MANION / 65 / BRADENTON, FLA.

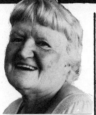

Doris Manion
65
Bradenton,
Fla.

"When I started my Easy Does It Yoga, my blood pressure was 140/80. After about six weeks of practice, when I went back to my doctor, **it had dropped to 124/80.**"

"**I feel it has made me stronger since I had my stroke.** I do my Yoga at home and I do feel better."

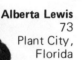

Alberta Lewis
73
Plant City,
Florida

"**I showed my doctor this book,** because I have a problem with my blood pressure. He told me to keep doing it easy, because since I've been exercising, it's been down to normal."

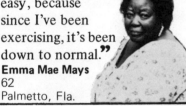

Emma Mae Mays
62
Palmetto, Fla.

"Because of my physical limitation, good blood circulation is a must and I get such a beautiful feeling from the exercise that I know when my circulation is working right or wrong. In fact, any of the exercises that require a little extra effort bring to me that lovely feeling in my head— I can actually feel the circulation and more oxygen in my brain by stretching. It

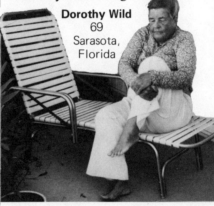

Dorothy Wild
69
Sarasota,
Florida

feels as though there's more oxygen in your brain, and it actually tingles. After my Yoga I tingle all over, as though I'm waking up. **That's how I know when my circulation's improved.**"

"**It feels good to get fresh blood up into your brains.** I even think this Yoga exercise has helped my hair to start growing back again. My mother's 92, and the last time I saw her, she thought sure I was wearing a rug!"

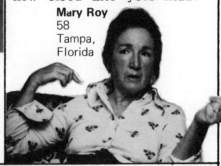

Gene Roy
62
Tampa,
Florida

"Gene used to be quite forgetful at times, but now he doesn't forget anything. In fact, he comes back with things from way back now. You know, I **think it has to do with getting new blood into your head!**"

Mary Roy
58
Tampa,
Florida

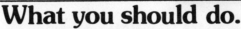
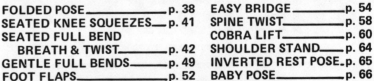

What you should do.

Some of the best exercises for improving your circulation are:

You should also look at the **nutritional suggestions on page 103,** and the **cautions and hints on page 95.**

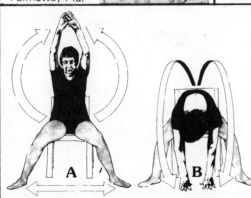

A   B

•ADDED YEARS•

"I HAD A GUN AND I WASN'T FAR FROM IT! I SAID 'WHAT IS THERE TO LIVE FOR...I'M ONLY GONNA END UP IMPOSING ON SOMEONE ELSE'."

GENE ROY / 62 / TAMPA, FLORIDA

Gene Roy
62
Tampa,
Florida

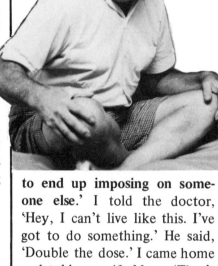

❝This Yoga was a blessing from God for me. I think that it gave me a few years on my life. Not only that, but a lot happier years without having that constant pain and drag. It was as though part of you was dead, but you're still moving I was going down fast—been through seven operations and was on 26 pills a day for pain and what not. Valium for depression—you name it. I was climbing the walls like a nut. **And I had a gun and I wasn't far from it! I said, 'What is there to live for? I'm only going to end up imposing on someone else.'** I told the doctor, 'Hey, I can't live like this. I've got to do something.' He said, 'Double the dose.' I came home and told my wife Mary, 'That's it.' I dumped all the pills in the toilet and flushed it. That was five years ago.

'I was so determined to be out of that condition that when I started this Yoga exercise there was some pain, sure, but nothing like what I'd already been through in those past years. Before this Yoga I never did any exercise at all. Now, hey, I feel so good. Everything's feeling so good! It's just like a new body. It's helped give me back 99¾% of my life. My God, I'm a new person. Not only that, but I'm more potent now. Ha! It helps you in more ways than one. **It's my Yoga—that's what I attribute the whole business to!"**

Annie Mae Johnson
63
Palmetto,
Florida

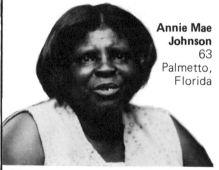

❝I think these exercises may keep you living a little longer and help you get around your hurts.❞

Jim Chesser
77
Dover, Florida

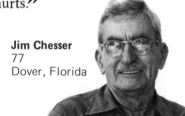

❝You can't just lay down and die! I don't have too much longer to live, but I want to live as good as I can be, as healthy as I can. I do all I can do!❞

What you should do.

THE TOTAL YOU
YOUR DAILY ROUTINE FOR TOTAL FITNESS

Turn directly to **Section 9, Daily Routines, on pages 95—100,** to learn how to put all aspects of Easy Does It Yoga into your life.

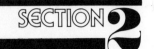
•MORE ENERGY & PEP•

"NOW I GO DISCO DANCING EVERY WEDNESDAY & THURSDAY."

JEANNE HROVAT / 66 / EUCLID, OHIO

"Doing this Yoga every day has made me a changed person. I feel so alive now that I just want to do things. I used to feel so dopey—you know, sluggish and fatigued. I just felt so sluggish that I'd just as soon lay on the davenport and just sleep or nap, rather than doing anything. NOW, oh heavens, you wouldn't believe what a changed person I am. **Now I go disco dancing every Wednesday and Thursday.** Not in my wildest dreams would I have thought that I would even have the energy to go out and do these things. It's just grand!"

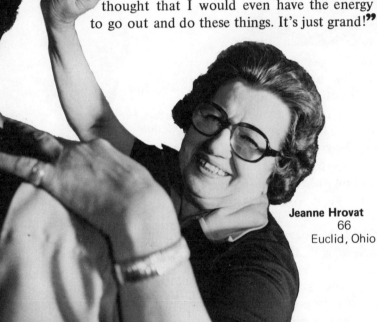

Jeanne Hrovat
66
Euclid, Ohio

"You know that Myrtis Weeks? Do you know before she started the Yoga exercises they'd have to bring her her tray from the lunch line. **Now she comes trotting down through the line like a 16 year old.**"

Peggie Sleda
67
Seffner, Florida

"This Yoga is the most exciting thing that has happened to me in my whole life." **Myrtis Weeks**
81
Seffner, Florid

"With this Yoga you just feel better. Not like an old dead log any more. Now I feel like a fish in water! Yeah, that Yoga, you keep up with it, **you aren't gonna sit down somewhere and just drop off into nothing.**"

John Alexander
70 Palmetto, Florida

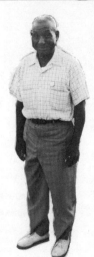

What you should do.

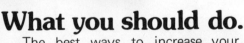

The best ways to increase your energy level are to **practice the breathing exercises in Section 7, pages 79—86.** You should also do the **Seated and Standing Full Bend Breath exercises on pages 42 and 49.** Improving your diet and **nutrition might also help: see pages 104—106.**

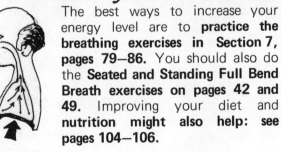

• MEDITATION HELPS •

"WHEN I GET REAL TENSE AND KEYED UP THE DEEP BREATHING & MEDITATION REALLY, REALLY HELP."

JOSEPHINE VIDMAR / 70 / CLEVELAND, OHIO

"My husband passed away ten years ago. I was depressed for a long time. **The Yoga and meditation seems to give me a different viewpoint about life and death.** You have to learn to accept things that are in God's hands. My Yoga gives me a tranquil feeling and somehow, you just feel relaxed and a whole lot happier and everything."

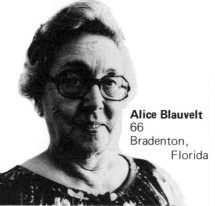

Alice Blauvelt
66
Bradenton,
Florida

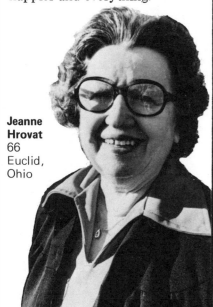

Jeanne Hrovat
66
Euclid,
Ohio

"I usually do my meditation around four o'clock in the afternoon. It's the time of day when everything is quiet around here. I turn the TV off and pull the blinds. **Four o'clock seems to be my best time. I use the meditation to help control my asthma.** Most of my asthma problems, and most of my problems in general, are caused by nerves and depression, and **I've noticed a big improvement in that area.** The biggest thing anybody with asthma can do is to relax so the meditation really helps me."

"And this isn't just some surface thing for right now like watching TV or a movie and then an hour from now you'll forget it. **This stays with you because it's something you can value the rest of your life.**"

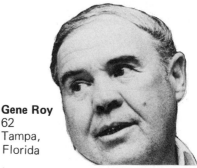

Gene Roy
62
Tampa,
Florida

"**The meditation is great,** especially when you completely relax. You relax your throat, your ankles, and everything. I find that tremendous."

Helen Gould
64
Euclid, Ohio

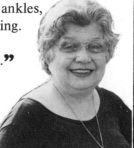

What you should do.

Your EDY exercises and breathing will help you to relax, but even more important are the **complete relaxation procedure** and **two meditation techniques** that can be done seated in a chair or lying on the floor. These can be found in **Section 8 on pages 87–94.**

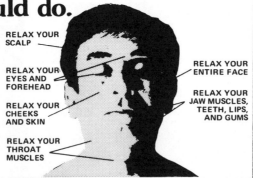

RELAX YOUR SCALP

RELAX YOUR EYES AND FOREHEAD

RELAX YOUR CHEEKS AND SKIN

RELAX YOUR THROAT MUSCLES

RELAX YOUR ENTIRE FACE

RELAX YOUR JAW MUSCLES, TEETH, LIPS, AND GUMS

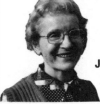

Josephine Vidmar
70
Cleveland, Ohio

"I have a lot of tension and pressure in my life. **When I get real tense and keyed up the deep breathing and meditation really really help.**"

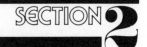

• DRIVING BETTER •

"BEFORE, I COULD NEVER TURN LIKE THIS TO LOOK OVER MY SHOULDER. NOW I CAN ACTUALLY TURN. IT'S UNBELIEVABLE!"

JEANNE HROVAT / 66 / EUCLID, OHIO

"It was very hard for me to get in and out of cars, even big ones. I always had to be helped—no, pulled out! Took me a long time getting in and out. **But now, since my Yoga, that problem's gone** because I can move now! I even drive better. When I'd be driving, I'd have to lean all the way over to see a little bit behind me. I had such a stiff neck. And you see my daughter, all she does is turn her head and glance. Now my Yoga's loosened me up so I am able to glance too. I thought it was the kind of glasses I was wearing that was the hindrance. Here it was because I was so stiff!"

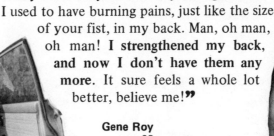

"I have arthritis in my back and neck so I could never turn when I was in the car. I always had to use the mirror to back up. **Since my Yoga, I can go all the way back, with my neck, like this!**"

Jeanne Hrovat
66
Euclid, Ohio

"I used to have to have a pillow behind my back to drive my car. After practicing this Yoga for some time my wife asked one day, 'Hey, where's your pillow?' I answered, 'What pillow? I don't need it any more.' My back is way stronger now. Why, I used to have burning pains, just like the size of your fist, in my back. Man, oh man, oh man! **I strengthened my back, and now I don't have them any more.** It sure feels a whole lot better, believe me!"

Gene Roy
62
Tampa,
Florida

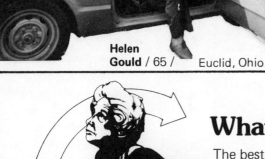

Helen Gould / 65 / Euclid, Ohio

What you should do:

The best poses for increasing flexibility in the spine are:

• FEELINGS OF WELL-BEING •

"I NEVER HAD A SENSE OF 'WELL-BEING', IN FACT, MOST DAYS I FELT REALLY BAD."

CHARLOTTE SHADE / 60 / LAND O'LAKES, FLORIDA

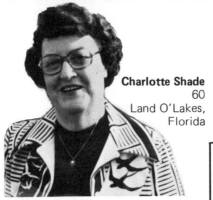

Charlotte Shade
60
Land O'Lakes,
Florida

"I have had a muscle problem for over 25 years which has kept me from doing many things, even many household chores. Some doctors said it was arthritis, but most doctors said they really didn't know what it was. They prescribed arthritis medicine and too much aspirin, from which I developed a gastric ulcer. My lower back and shoulders have been in constant pain, and my muscles ached all over and were sore to the touch. I never had a sense of 'well-being'; in fact, most days I felt really bad. I always felt inside that exercise might help, but not one doctor ever encouraged me. In fact, most even discouraged me. Eventually, I started an exercise routine of my own. They did help me for a while, but I couldn't keep it up for any length of time because the ones I picked were too strenuous. However, I have now been practicing Easy Does It Yoga for over three months, and the change is remarkable. I am no longer afraid to move for fear of muscle spasms, and my muscles feel much stronger. The pain in my lower back is completely gone, and the pain between my shoulders only returns if I overdo with my arms. This also is getting better. The pain used to be constant, nagging, and often very severe. But now, it's relieved. I'm much more flexible. I have more energy and I am actually participating in life again, and it's great. I know I've got to be regular in my routine to maintain and improve my progress, **but it's really** wonderful to know that by doing this Easy Does It Yoga, that I have a chance to feel better than I have in years. I find life exciting again and good. And my husband thinks I'm much more fun to be with!"

"My Yoga leads to a general feeling of 'well-being.' As my strength and control of my body has improved, I have a feeling of 'physical well-being'

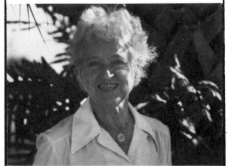

Harriet Peel / 74 Sarasota, Florida

which gives impetus to a greater participation in recreational and social activities. My family and friends have commented favorably on the change in my personal appearance. This gives a lift to one's mental outlook which, in turn, results in a feeling of 'emotional well-being.' The Yoga philosophy and meditation also leads to a 'spiritual well-being,' and self-acceptance —an acceptance of one's own years and that we are worthwhile, with contributions yet to make in life."

What you should do.

THE TOTAL YOU
YOUR DAILY ROUTINE FOR TOTAL FITNESS

Turn directly to the **Total You Routine on page 97,** in **Section 9, Daily Routines,** and be sure to practice the **5 Ways to Increase Personal Growth on page 111.**

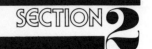

"AS LONG AS I'M ABLE TO HELP MYSELF, I'LL FEEL BETTER ABOUT MYSELF."

SAM ODUM / 72 / PALMETTO, FLORIDA

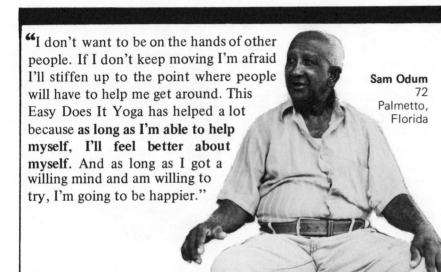

"I don't want to be on the hands of other people. If I don't keep moving I'm afraid I'll stiffen up to the point where people will have to help me get around. This Easy Does It Yoga has helped a lot because **as long as I'm able to help myself, I'll feel better about myself.** And as long as I got a willing mind and am willing to try, I'm going to be happier."

Sam Odum
72
Palmetto,
Florida

"My Yoga interest is the first time in my life that I did something for myself— for me alone."

Harriet Peel
74
Sarasota,
Florida

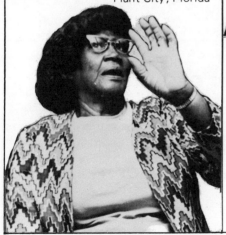

"Last week I actually reached up and painted my awnings and house myself. I hadn't been able to do something like that for a long time. But since my Yoga, I just reached right up there and didn't even get sore from all that stretching and craning my neck. **I did it all myself!**"

Dora Richardson / 70
Plant City, Florida

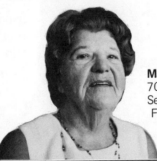

"If people would take exercise regularly as they get older, **they would be better able to take care of themselves.**"

Mae Tyus
70
Seffner,
Florida

**Dorothy
Wild**
69
Sarasota,
Florida

"Since my physical limitations have curtailed most of my activities, I really have a psychological need to feel like I'm accomplishing something or I get despondent and depressed. **Improving my physical abilities in my Yoga helps give me that needed sense of accomplishment.**"

What you should do.

Independence depends upon your mobility. The best exercises for your legs are:

You should also read and put into practice the concepts in **Section 11, Philosophy, pages 108–111.**

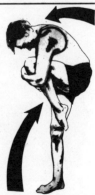

• MORE AWARE & ALERT •

"ALL OF A SUDDEN I SEEM MORE AWARE. IT'S THE CRAZIEST THING."

DORIS MANION / 65 / BRADENTON, FLORIDA

"It's made me more alert. It seems like I get more air, more energy, and everybody's remarking about how much more alert I seem and they all wish they could be like me."

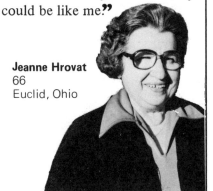

Jeanne Hrovat
66
Euclid, Ohio

"I do my meditation and breathing regularly, and you know, I think my concentration is a lot better, because I'm more aware of things. It's hard to explain, but I noticed it first while driving. It used to be that I never paid much attention to where I was going. But **all of a sudden I seem more aware. It's the craziest thing.** I notice the street signs and where I'm going. It used to be that I just didn't care, but now I'm taking an interest in things that I never would have before. It's strange. I think, 'Why am I noticing that? I've gone by here a hundred times, but now it's all new to me!'"

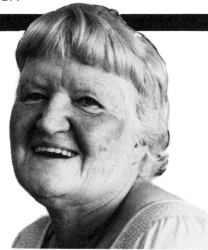

Doris Manion / 65 / Bradenton, Fla.

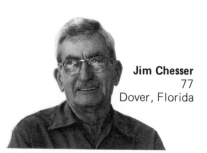

Jim Chesser
77
Dover, Florida

"It's helped me be more alert, and I think people understand me better."

"You can make yourself sick just by thinking, and a lot of these older people today, they get so despondent they just quit living. But not me—I got it—I get the benefit of this Yoga. Just don't overdo, that's all. Don't overdo. **Build up slowly and keep going, and sure enough you'll be compensated for your efforts. And you'll feel more alive.**"

Gene Roy / 62 / Tampa, Florida

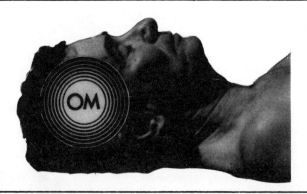

What you should do.

To learn how to meditate, turn to **pages 87–94, Section 8: Relaxation and Meditation.** Also look at the diet suggestions for confusion and anemia on page 104 and be sure to read the **5 Ways to Increase Personal Growth** on **page 111.**

"I SLEEP BETTER IF I DO MY DEEP BREATHING EVERY DAY."

HELEN GOULD / 65 / EUCLID, OHIO

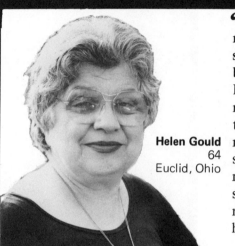

Helen Gould
64
Euclid, Ohio

"The deep breathing has helped me to relax tremendously. **I sleep better if I do my deep breathing every day.** Sometimes I used to go for four or five nights with very little sleep, that's murder. I was getting really depressed from a lack of sleep. But now my Yoga relaxes me so much that I not only sleep better at night, but I can nap in the afternoon, which I hadn't been able to do in years."

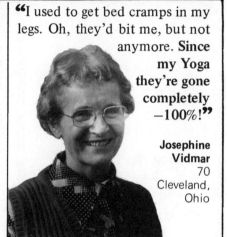

"I used to get bed cramps in my legs. Oh, they'd bit me, but not anymore. Since my Yoga they're gone completely –100%!"

Josephine Vidmar
70
Cleveland, Ohio

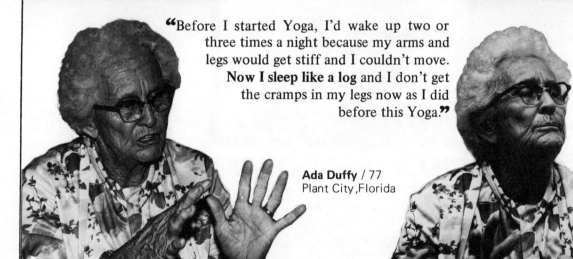

"Before I started Yoga, I'd wake up two or three times a night because my arms and legs would get stiff and I couldn't move. **Now I sleep like a log** and I don't get the cramps in my legs now as I did before this Yoga."

Ada Duffy / 77
Plant City, Florida

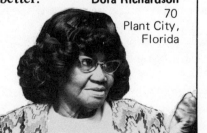

"It's even helped me to sleep better." **Dora Richardson**
70
Plant City, Florida

What you should do:

If you suffer from insomnia, you need to learn the **Relaxing Breath on page 86,** as well as the other breathing exercises in **Section 7, pages 79–86.** You should also practice the **Complete Relaxation Procedure on pages 89–90,** and see **page 104** for **Nutrition Hints.**

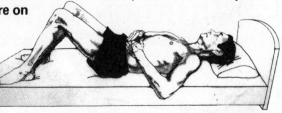

HOW TO USE
THIS
BOOK

> "Oh, this is such a marvelous book. When I started out, I never did an exercise until I sat down and read it thoroughly and concentrated on it. I keep it open next to me—like when I'm doing exercises—some place where I can read it and see if I'm doing it right. It's wonderful."
>
> **Maureen Ruth** / 73 / Bradenton, Florida

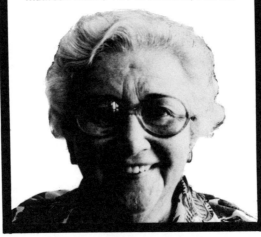

How do I begin?

The first thing you should do before actually beginning to practice is browse through the book and familiarize yourself with the way the book is designed.

You will notice as you review the book that Easy Does It Yoga is divided into five distinct but interrelated types of practice.

1 YOGA EXERCISES SECTION 3,4,5,6

These sections show you specially designed Yoga exercises almost anyone can do regardless of any physical limitations. These exercises can be done in a chair, standing, on the floor, in a wheelchair, in a bed, and in the bathtub. In Section 6 you will also find eye exercises and massage procedures.

2 BREATHING EXERCISES SECTION 7

In this section you'll learn all about your breathing, how it works, and how to recognize and correct poor breathing habits through simple daily Yoga breathing exercises.

3 RELAXATION & MEDITATION SECTION 8

This section teaches you a complete relaxation procedure and two meditation techniques which can be practiced while lying down or seated in a chair.

4 NUTRITION SECTION 10

In this section you'll learn how to improve your health by modifying your eating habits and inexpensively improving your nutrition.

5 PHILOSOPHY SECTION 11

This section teaches you about the philosophical foundation of Easy Does It Yoga and gives you five ways to increase your personal growth and find greater meaning and purpose in your life.

● SECTION HEADERS & NUMBERS

As you look through the book, notice that in the upper right- and left-hand corners of each page there is a section number and title. This will allow you to easily find the exercise or technique you are looking for.

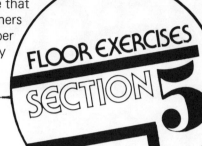

● THE SPIRAL BINDING

The spiral binding of your book is an important part of its design. It will allow the book to lie flat on the floor or table next to you.

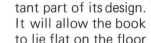

● CLEAR STEP-BY-STEP ILLUSTRATION

The hundreds of large step-by-step illustrations and photographs graphically show you exactly what each technique and exercise looks like before you try to do it.

● USE IT WHILE YOU PRACTICE

Most importantly, this book has been carefully designed to help you as you actually practice Easy Does It Yoga. Keep it next to you as you do the various techniques so that you can check yourself against the illustration and readily refer to the instructional copy.

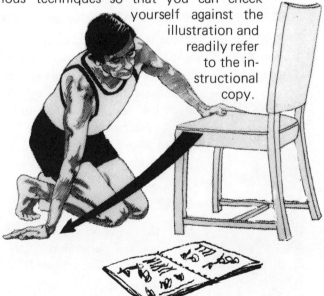

Which section should I start with to actually begin practicing?

After you have looked through the book and read some of the things that interest you, then you're ready to begin to practice. In order to start working with the book, turn to Section 9, Daily Routines, on page 95. In this section you will learn helpful cautions and hints and a step-by-step daily and weekly program that will start you off gently and safely in your Easy Does It Yoga practice.

EASY DOES IT YOGA
EXERCISES

Easy Does It Yoga exercise is not just for your body. It is designed to also increase your energy levels, awareness, concentration, and mind/body coordination. Each exercise you will learn will involve the following three areas:

BODY ———— BREATH ———— MIND

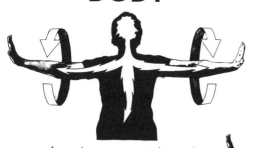

BREATH
All of life's movements, even mental thought, depend upon the subtle energy and power of breath. Hence the quality, depth, and control of breathing accompanies Yoga exercise in specific ways.

MIND
In Yoga the aim is not just physical health but, even more importantly, mental health becomes the goal. Specific mental methods of observation are utilized while you exercise in order to enhance clarity of mind and awareness.

BODY
In order to move and exercise the body, the brain must send nerve impulses through the nerve pathways and stimulate muscles. The muscles then contract and move the body.

Many standard fitness programs developed for the average American have discouraged older people because they are either too difficult and painful, or too childish and boring. Nothing is more embarrassing than walking into a roomful of youngsters doing push-ups when you're incapable of getting up and down off the floor. On the other hand, Maggie Kuhn, president of the Grey Panthers, talks about the demeaning position of "being treated like a baby with wrinkles." A back-slapping fitness director, who treats you as if you were an imbecile, can rob you of all motivation for exercising.

The EDY program avoids these pitfalls because it is engaging and challenging, and at the same time lets you work within your own limitations. These exercises can be done by the most frail, bedridden elderly student, and yet can also inspire the older fitness buff.

Because EDY exercise is a new and different approach, people look forward to practicing it every day. The program is not boring because it is progressive. In addition, because it involves every muscle group in the body, specific breathing patterns and mental concentration, it is successful where other fitness programs may have been ineffective.

The EDY exercises can be done without any expensive ___t or special environment. You can do these ___ seated on a chair, in the bathtub or ___hed, in a wheelchair, and even ___u no longer have the excuse ___ak, tired, busy, or afraid to

Easy Does It Yoga exercise brings about
TOTAL FITNESS
through the development of
**Better Functioning Brain & Nerves
Improved Circulation
Strong, Limber Muscles & Joints
Healthier Vital Organs**

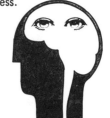

"At my age, I thought that I was just too old for Yoga. I've gone to lots of exercise classes at spas and other places, but they really don't understand that I can't do a lot of the strenuous things they want me to do. I might not notice the strain at the time, but the next day, watch out! This Yoga is nice and easy, and that's why I like it so much. I guess that's why you call it 'Easy Does It'."

Mae Norris / 84 / Seffner, Fla.

CHAIR EXERCISES SECTION 3

Of the thousands of older people we have worked with, the majority are usually a bit reluctant to begin exercising for two reasons: one is that many of them have not exercised for years; and the other is that they are just plain frightened of the word exercise. For this reason, your Easy Does It Yoga exercises begin in a chair. Also, you will notice that throughout the exercise sections we have included helpful massage procedures that will not only help you exercise, but relieve stiffness and soreness as well.

SHOULDER SHRUGS

The easiest way to begin exercising is to strengthen and loosen up your shoulders. 1. Sit up straight and lift your shoulders up and back as far as possible. **2.** Roll your shoulders forward, and then relax them down. **3.** When done correctly, your shoulders should go in a circular motion. This exercise can be done in circles both forward and backward. Repeat 3—5 times.

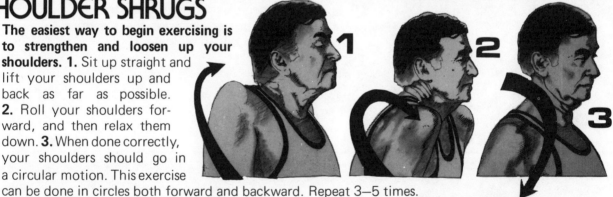

SINGLE SHOULDER SHRUG

Do 3—5 shoulder shrugs forward and 3—5 backwards with your right shoulder; then do the same number with your left shoulder. As you get stronger, increase rotations to 5—10 each way.

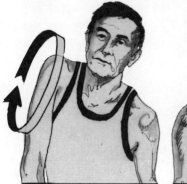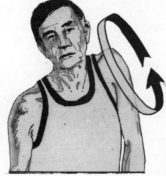

DOUBLE SHOULDER SHRUG

After you do your single shoulder rotations, rest a minute; then do both shoulders at once. Do 3—5 rotations forward, and 3 — 5 backwards. Move slowly and gently in circular motions and don't strain. After a few weeks you'll notice greater limberness and strength.

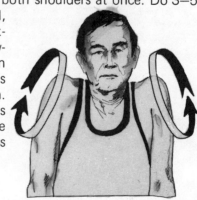

ELBOW ROLLS

The Elbow Rolls exercise is an easy way to loosen stiff shoulder joints as well as strengthen all muscles of the shoulders and neck.

Sit up straight and lift your elbows up, as in the illustration. Now simply rotate your elbows slowly, making large circles.

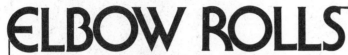
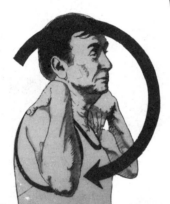

Do 5 rotations forward, then 5 rotations backwards. As you get stronger and more limber, increase the rotations to 10 forward, 10 backwards.

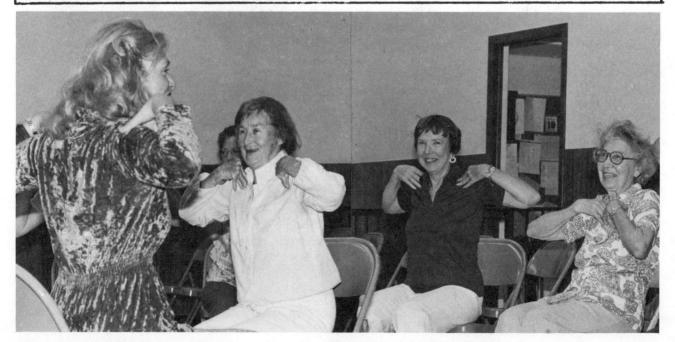

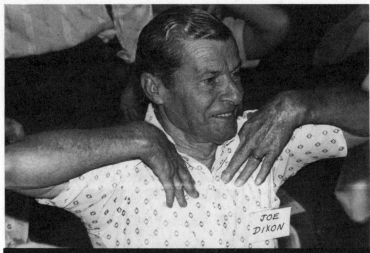

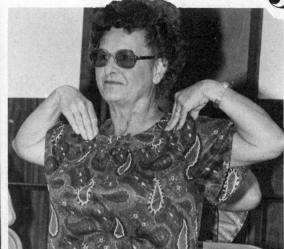

"I had a pain in my shoulder... it was like an icepick. This is the exercise that really helped."

Gene Roy
62
Tampa, Florida

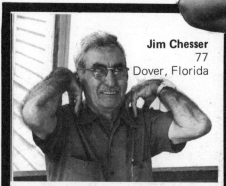

Jim Chesser
77
Dover, Florida

"This Yoga helped me quite a bit. I got arthritis in my hips, legs and hands and all. It's just stiff to move, you know. It hurt to move. **By doing this Yoga exercise, it helps you get limbered up,** and I can bend over more. I can even walk a little better without so much pain."

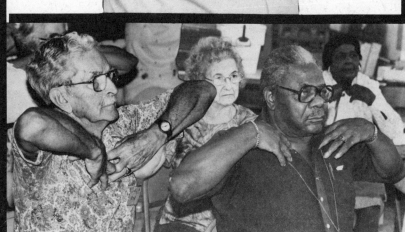

35

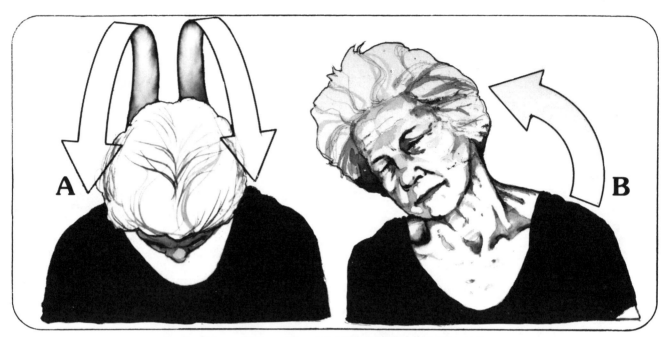

HEAD ROTATIONS

Sit comfortably in a chair, keeping the spine erect and your hands resting on your knees. Now, simply lower your chin toward your chest **(A).** Then lower your right ear toward your right shoulder **(B).** Next drop your head backward gently **(C).** Then lower your left ear toward your left shoulder **(D). Remember: Do not strain. This exercise is designed to limber the neck and relieve tension. Continue from one position to the next in a gentle, circular fashion. Then stop and go in the opposite direction a few times. Do not snap the head. This is to be done very slowly and gently. You can also do this exercise standing with your arms raised out to the side, parallel to the floor with the palms up.**

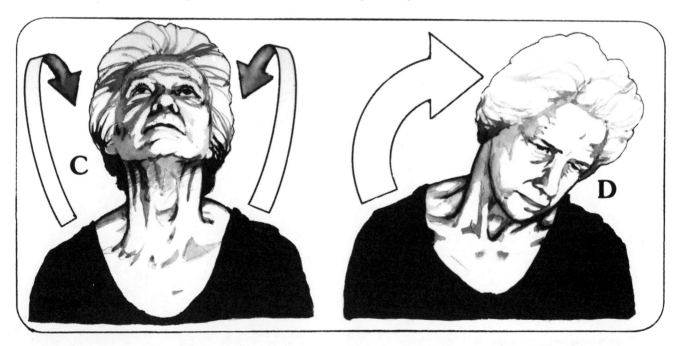

ARM REACHES

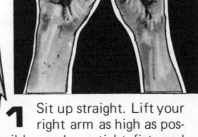

Many people suffer from stiff, sore shoulders. These arm exercises may help alleviate this discomfort.

1 Sit up straight. Lift your right arm as high as possible, make a tight fist and look up at your hand, holding this position for a moment. Then relax and lower your arm. Repeat 3—5 times with each arm.

2 Then do the same exercise with both arms at once. Repeat 3—5 times with both arms. **NOTE: After doing this series of arm and shoulder exercises, you may want to do the shoulder and arm massage in Section 6.**

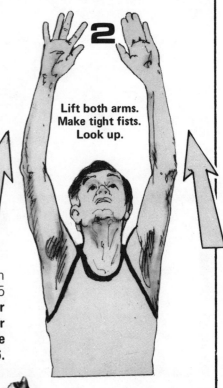

Lift both arms. Make tight fists. Look up.

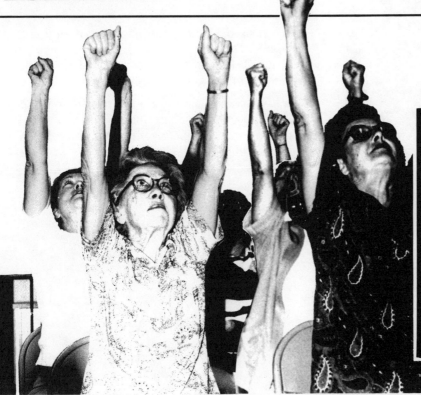

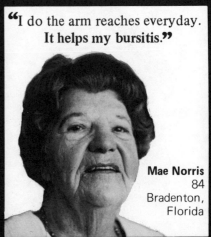

"I do the arm reaches everyday. It helps my bursitis."

Mae Norris
84
Bradenton, Florida

ARM ROTATIONS

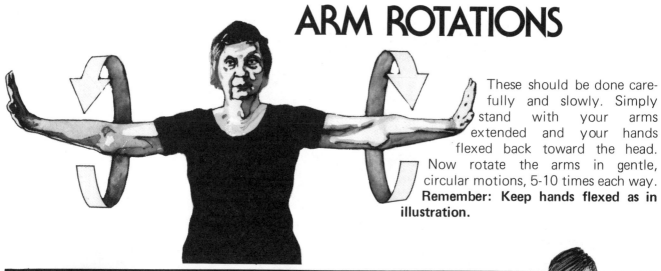

These should be done carefully and slowly. Simply stand with your arms extended and your hands flexed back toward the head. Now rotate the arms in gentle, circular motions, 5-10 times each way. **Remember: Keep hands flexed as in illustration.**

SHOULDER & ELBOW MASSAGE

It is helpful to get in the habit of massaging your shoulders, elbows, etc. either before or after your exercises. This will increase the benefits of your exercising and you'll love it! See page 75

FOLDED POSE

This is the beginning exercise to help you get used to bending over without the dizziness or fear that so many people suffer from.

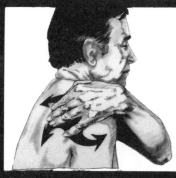

Breathe in

Breathe out

1 The first step is to put your hands on your knees or thighs and breathe out as you bend forward. Then breathe in and come back up to **Position 2. Repeat this procedure 3—5 times, slowly breathing in and out through the nose.**

3 Afterwards simply fold in half in your lap and wrap your arms around your legs. Focus your attention exclusively on your breathing, and each time you exhale, relax more and more.

Relax your breathing more and more.

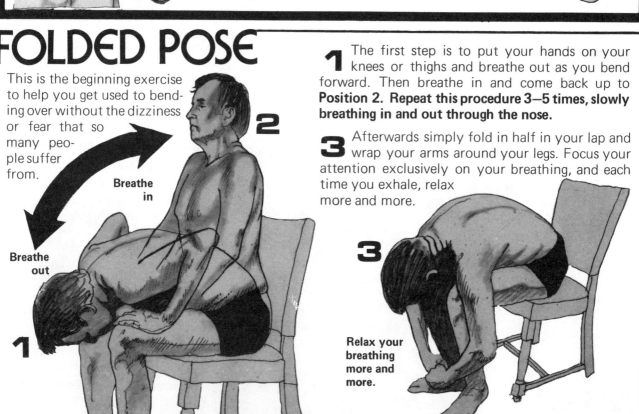

38

ELBOW TO KNEE

Both of these exercises are great for limbering up, but make sure you breathe correctly.

1 Sit up straight, clasp your hands behind your head, and breathe in deeply.

2 Then breathe out as you bend and twist towards your right knee with your left elbow.

3 Come right back up to **Position 1** as you breathe in and then breathe out again, bending and twisting to your left knee with your right elbow. **Remember: Breathe deeply through the nose. Bend and twist slowly. Repeat 3—5 times to each knee.**

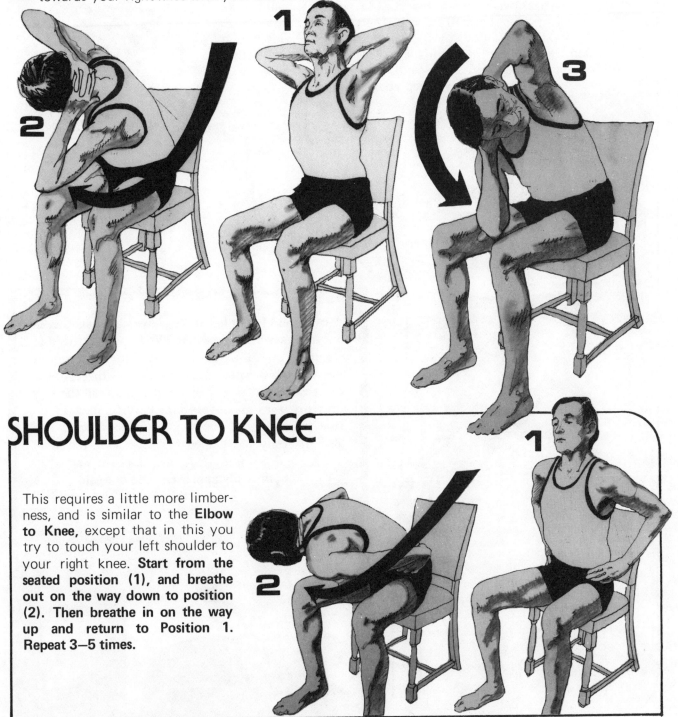

SHOULDER TO KNEE

This requires a little more limberness, and is similar to the **Elbow to Knee,** except that in this you try to touch your left shoulder to your right knee. **Start from the seated position (1), and breathe out on the way down to position (2). Then breathe in on the way up and return to Position 1. Repeat 3—5 times.**

SEATED TWIST

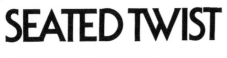

Sit comfortably in a straight-backed chair. Do not lean against the chairback; rather, sit slightly forward. First, take your right hand and place it on your left knee. Place your left hand behind you on the chair seat. Now gently twist to the left, looking back over your left shoulder **(A).** Hold this position,, breathing gently for about 10 seconds. Then relax, turn forward and repeat the exercise to the right. Repeat this process 3 times in each direction. **Remember: Do not lift legs. Keep them forward with the feet flat on the floor. Twist gently as far as possible. Move slowly. Keep your eyes open.**

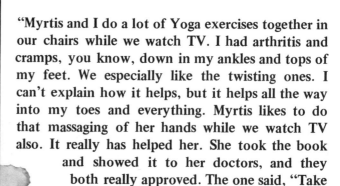

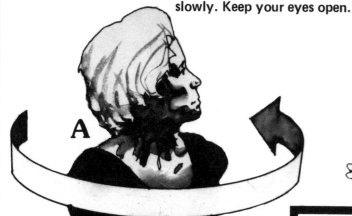

"Myrtis and I do a lot of Yoga exercises together in our chairs while we watch TV. I had arthritis and cramps, you know, down in my ankles and tops of my feet. We especially like the twisting ones. I can't explain how it helps, but it helps all the way into my toes and everything. Myrtis likes to do that massaging of her hands while we watch TV also. It really has helped her. She took the book and showed it to her doctors, and they both really approved. The one said, "Take this home and use it!""

Willard Weeks / 79
Seffner,
Florida

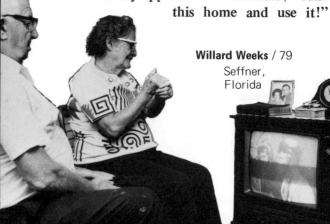

40

SEATED LEG LIFT

Grasp the chair seat with the hands. Straighten the right leg. Breathe in slowly lifting the leg straight up as high as possible, then lower the leg to the floor as you exhale. Repeat this with the opposite leg. Do 3-7 repetitions with each leg.

"It's the knee lifts that helped me the most. I know my Yoga does me good because my knee has always bothered me. I have arthritis in my knee, but it's lots better now. I haven't been having the pains very much. In fact, I haven't had much pain all this week, and none last week. It's been doing real good."

Agnes Barton / 64
Fairfield, Florida

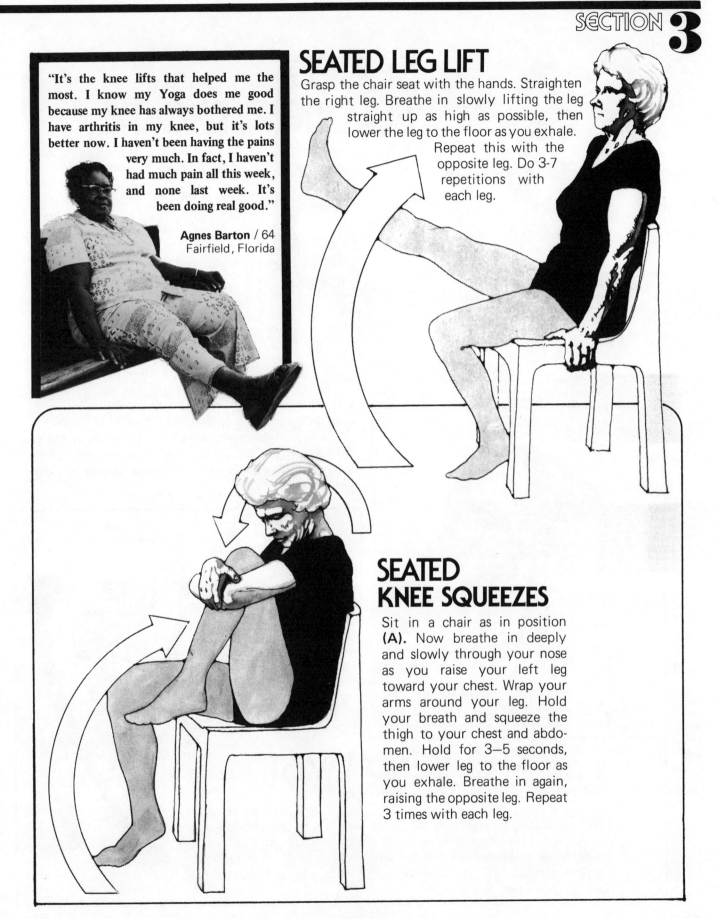

SEATED KNEE SQUEEZES

Sit in a chair as in position **(A).** Now breathe in deeply and slowly through your nose as you raise your left leg toward your chest. Wrap your arms around your leg. Hold your breath and squeeze the thigh to your chest and abdomen. Hold for 3—5 seconds, then lower leg to the floor as you exhale. Breathe in again, raising the opposite leg. Repeat 3 times with each leg.

SEATED FULL BEND BREATH

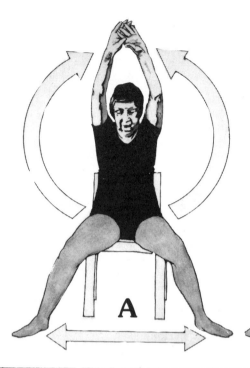

Sit forward on your chair so that you are not leaning on the chair back. Spread your legs as far back as is comfortable **(A).** Breathe in slowly and deeply through the nose as you raise your arms over the head. Then slowly exhale as you bend forward and stretch out toward the floor **(B).** Ideally, both hands should touch the floor. However, reach as far as you can without straining. Pause for a moment in this position, then breathe in slowly as you raise up with the arms overhead **(A).** Then exhale, lowering your arms to the legs and relax. Repeat this process 3-5 times. **Remember: Breathe through your nose. Breathe deeply and slowly, filling and emptying the lungs completely. Breathe and raise slowly in time with the breathing.**

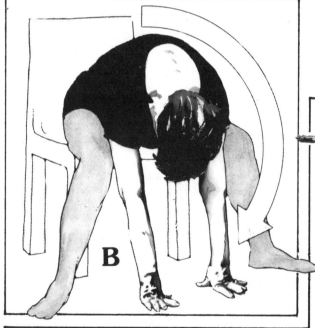

Look up at your hand and hold this position for a moment.

FULL BEND TWIST

1 Sit up straight. Spread your legs apart 2—3 feet, as in **Position 1.**

2 After you breathe in deeply, then breathe out as you bend and reach for your right foot with your left hand. As you do this, lift your right hand up and back, twisting as far as comfortable. Hold this position for a moment, looking at your hand. Then breathe in as you come back up to **Position 1. Repeat three times to each foot.**

STANDING EXERCISES
SECTION 4

"The only time I stand up is when I'm going somewhere else to either sit down or lie down."

The fact is, many older people have difficulty standing, and if forced to stand in lines for any length of time, may experience dizziness, weakness in the knees, loss of balance, and may even faint. The exercises in Section 4 will help to strengthen the muscles and nerves in your legs as well as the postural muscles that help you stand, walk, and generally get around better.

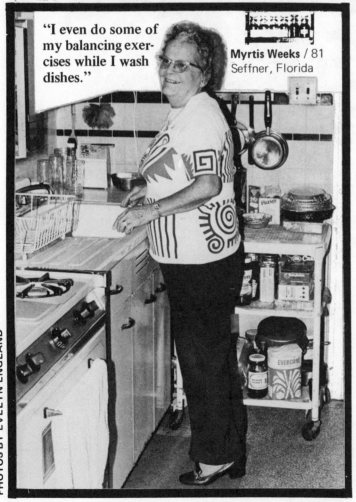

"I even do some of my balancing exercises while I wash dishes."

Myrtis Weeks / 81
Seffner, Florida

PHOTOS BY EVELYN ENGLAND

STANDING REACHES

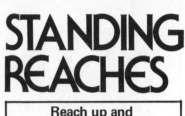

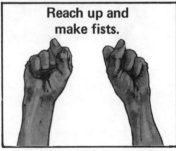

Reach up and make fists.

This exercise is just like the Arm Reaches done in a chair, except that you are standing on your toes.

Breathe in deeply through your nose and raise up on your toes. Hold your breath in as you hold the postion, making fists. Look up at your hands and stretch towards the ceiling. Hold for 3—5 seconds. Then exhale, and bring your arms down slowly to your sides and your feet to the floor. Repeat 3 times.

43

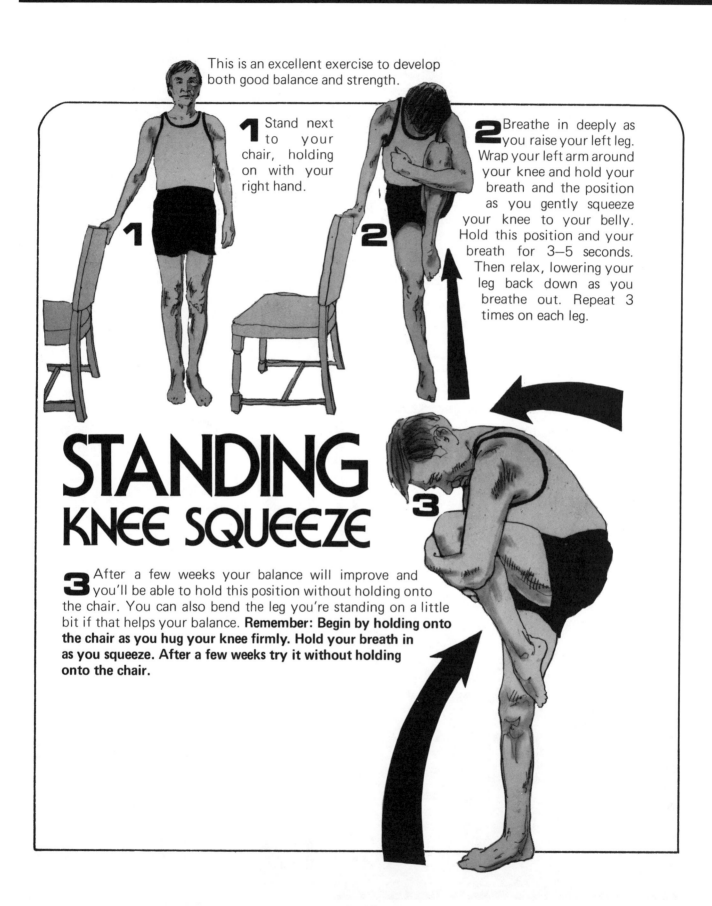

This is an excellent exercise to develop both good balance and strength.

1 Stand next to your chair, holding on with your right hand.

2 Breathe in deeply as you raise your left leg. Wrap your left arm around your knee and hold your breath and the position as you gently squeeze your knee to your belly. Hold this position and your breath for 3–5 seconds. Then relax, lowering your leg back down as you breathe out. Repeat 3 times on each leg.

STANDING KNEE SQUEEZE

3 After a few weeks your balance will improve and you'll be able to hold this position without holding onto the chair. You can also bend the leg you're standing on a little bit if that helps your balance. **Remember: Begin by holding onto the chair as you hug your knee firmly. Hold your breath in as you squeeze. After a few weeks try it without holding onto the chair.**

REAR ARM LIFTS

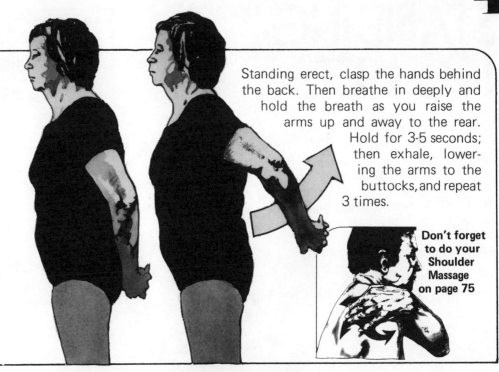

Standing erect, clasp the hands behind the back. Then breathe in deeply and hold the breath as you raise the arms up and away to the rear. Hold for 3-5 seconds; then exhale, lowering the arms to the buttocks, and repeat 3 times.

Don't forget to do your Shoulder Massage on page 75

TIP TOE BREATH

Stand erect with your arms as in Position **(A)**. Exhale, and then begin to inhale slowly and deeply, filling the lungs through the nose as you raise up off the floor on your toes **(B)**. Make fists with your hands and press in gently on the abdomen as you hold the position and the breath for 3—5 seconds; then exhale slowly, lowering the heels to the floor and your arms to the sides. Repeat 3 times.

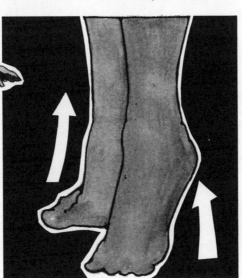

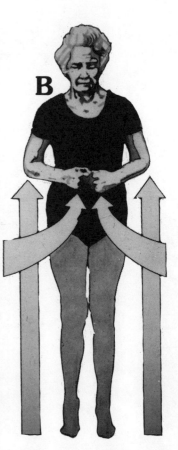

A

B

STANDING LEG LIFTS

Standing erect and holding onto the back of a chair to help your balance, slowly lift the left leg straight up in front of you as high as possible. Hold it for a moment; then lower it to the floor. Next, raise the leg directly to the side. Hold and lower. Repeat 3 times to the front and 3 times to the side with each leg.

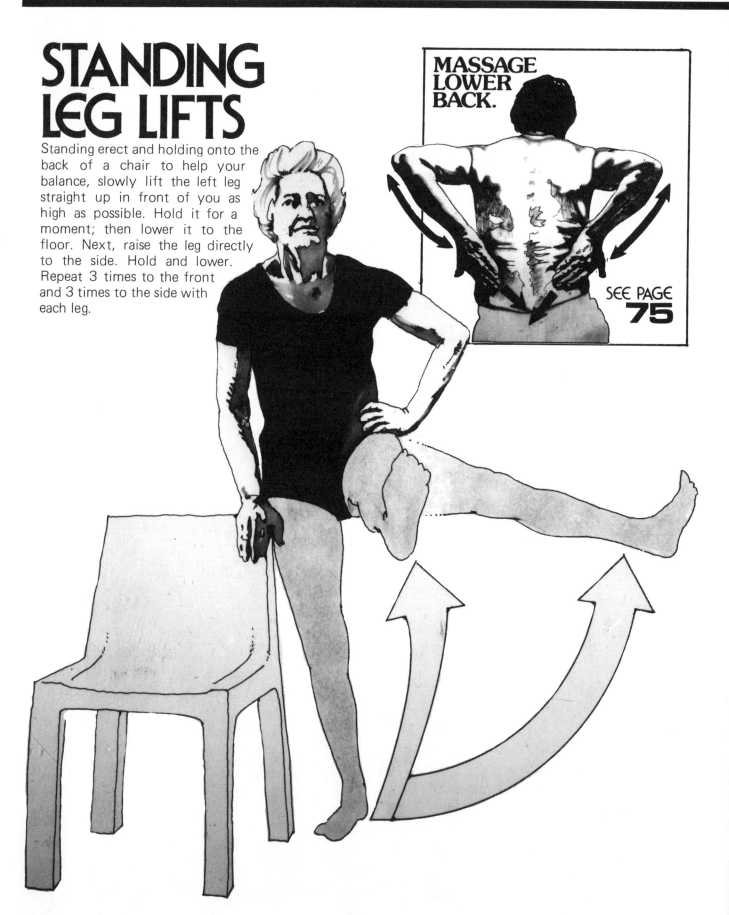

MASSAGE LOWER BACK.

SEE PAGE 75

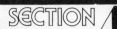

"I used to be real stiff and crippled up. The arthritis settled in the front of my legs all the way down to my toes. It got so that I couldn't lift my feet. So I had to slide them across the floor in order to get around. Now since my Yoga leg exercises I can not only lift my feet, but I can move my whole leg and get around by myself again."

Emma Mae Mays / 62
Palmetto, Florida

After you have practiced the Leg Lifts for a few weeks, try to bring the back leg up so that it is parallel to the floor and then slowly let go of the chair. Make sure that your body is parallel to the floor and look up between your hands.

REAR LEG LIFTS

SUPER BALANCE POSE

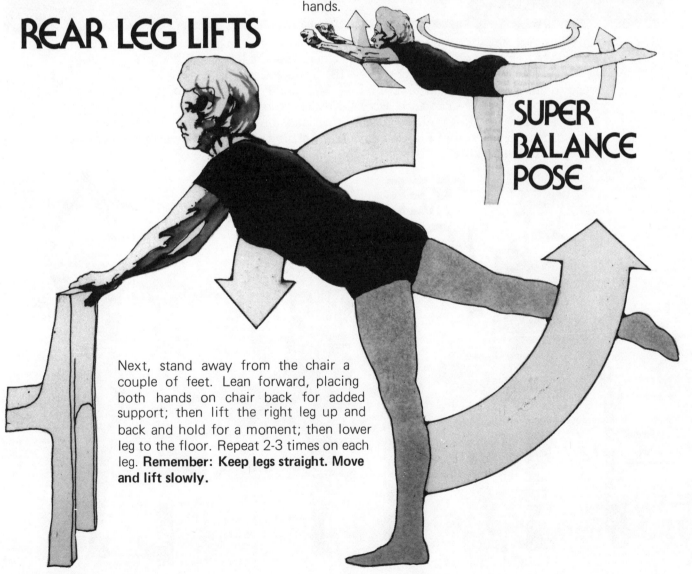

Next, stand away from the chair a couple of feet. Lean forward, placing both hands on chair back for added support; then lift the right leg up and back and hold for a moment; then lower leg to the floor. Repeat 2-3 times on each leg. **Remember: Keep legs straight. Move and lift slowly.**

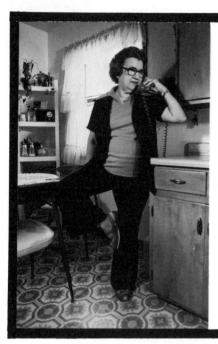

"Even when I'm on the telephone with one of my long-winded lady friends—ha!—I do my toe balances or leg raises or balancing exercises. They say, 'Hey, what are you doing.' I say, 'Never mind, go on!' I'm getting all my exercise, and they're just sitting!"

Jeanne Hrovat
66
Euclid, Ohio

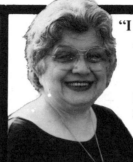

"I can stand on one foot and put on my socks now instead of holding onto a chair for balance. And I can do that tree pose with my foot way up on my leg. At 64, I think that's quite an accomplishment!"

Helen Gould
64 / Euclid, Ohio

"I have more confidence in myself because I got to where I don't have to hang onto the chair when I do my balance exercises."

Ruby Allen
87
Plant City, Florida

This exercise helps develop concentration, balance, and a healthy, strong nervous system. **(A)** Holding onto the back of the chair, raise the left leg up and place the foot carefully on the side of the right knee. **(B)** Raise the left hand slowly overhead and steady your balance. **(C)** Pick a spot on the floor about 6 feet in front of you and stare at it. This will help you balance. Now slowly let go of the chair and raise your right arm overhead. Hold this position for 10-30 seconds breathing gently. Then repeat the same process on the other leg. **Remember: Move slowly, maintaining balance. Stare at one spot. Breathe gently.**

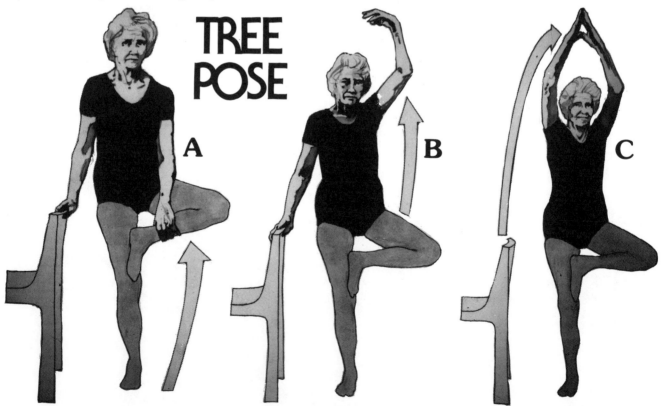

TREE POSE

A   B   C

"My forward bending exercises are a must every day. They do a lot for my circulation. When I bend over I can actually feel the fresh blood rushing down into my fingertips and back up into my arms."

Josephine Vidmar
70
Cleveland, Ohio

GENTLE FULL BENDS

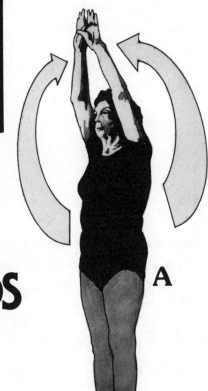

A

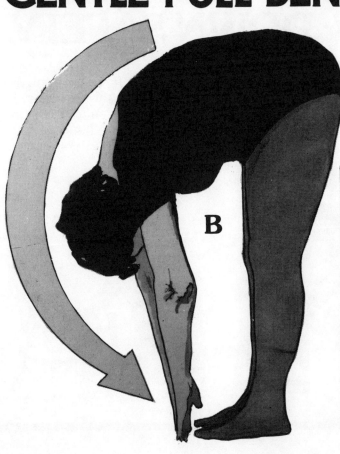

B

This is a little more advanced and can be tried after you get more limber. Standing erect with your feet about an inch apart, begin to breathe in, raising your arms overhead **(A)**. Now breathe out slowly as you bend and try to reach the floor **(B).** You must breathe deeply and fully in this exercise, and the legs must remain straight. Reach as far as you can toward the floor; then begin to breathe in, raising back up to Position **(A)**. Repeat 3–5 times. **Remember: Breathe deeply. Do not bend the legs. Reach as far as you can; eventually you will touch the floor. Move slowly and in a very relaxed manner.**

FLOOR EXERCISES
SECTION 5

Many people are afraid of getting down on the floor because they are afraid of injuring themselves or are afraid that they won't be able to get back up. This makes them feel awkward and also inhibits any idea of exercising on the floor. However, if you follow this simple, safe procedure, you will learn very quickly and easily how to get up and down anywhere. You will then be able to do the floor exercises every day.

Your Easy Does It Yoga technique for GETTING UP & DOWN SAFELY.

1 Stand in front of your chair, bend at the waist, and grasp the edge of your chair, supporting yourself. Make sure your chair is secure and won't slip.

2 Use your arms and the chair to support your weight. Bend your legs, lowering your right knee slowly and gently to the floor. Do only one knee at a time, starting with your right knee.

3 After your right knee is firmly on the floor you can then lower your left knee, but continue to hang onto the chair for support. Now you should be in a kneeling position, hanging onto your chair.

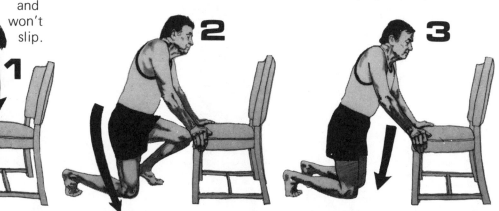

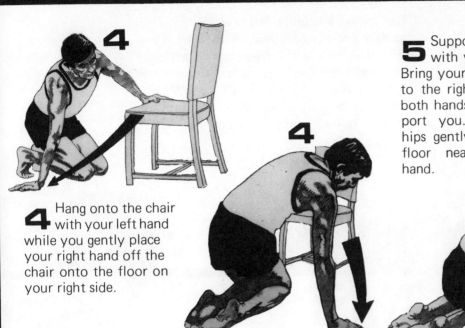

4 Hang onto the chair with your left hand while you gently place your right hand off the chair onto the floor on your right side.

5 Support your weight with your right arm. Bring your left hand over to the right also so that both hands and arms support you. Lower your hips gently down to the floor near your right hand.

6 Support yourself with your hands and arms. Lean back slightly, raising your left leg straight out in front of you.

7 Then unfold your right leg and straighten it out alongside your left leg. You should now be sitting on the floor with both legs in front, leaning on your arms.

GETTING BACK UP AGAIN...

In order to get back up again, simply get on your hands and knees in front of your chair, **Position 3.** Then raise your left leg up to **Position 2.** Push up with your arms and legs and stand right up slowly. At first practice steps **1, 2,** and **3** several times, getting up and down. Then go on to steps **4, 5, 6,** and **7.** Practice the whole process several times in order to get familiar with the procedure.

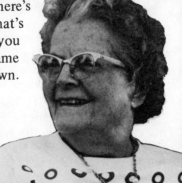

"That way of getting up and down is really great. My friends wanted to know how to do it, so I said, 'I'll show you how easy it is. It's just a matter of putting your legs and hands in the right place!' I showed them how, and they said, 'Well, there's nothing to it! That's really easy!' And you come up the same way you went down. **It's great!"**

Myrtis Weeks
81
Seffner, Florida

51

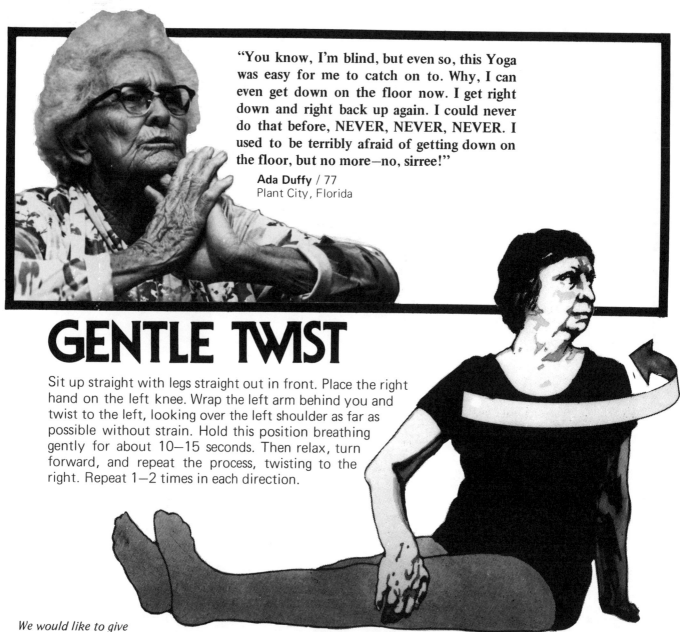

"You know, I'm blind, but even so, this Yoga was easy for me to catch on to. Why, I can even get down on the floor now. I get right down and right back up again. I could never do that before, NEVER, NEVER, NEVER. I used to be terribly afraid of getting down on the floor, but no more—no, sirree!"

Ada Duffy / 77
Plant City, Florida

GENTLE TWIST

Sit up straight with legs straight out in front. Place the right hand on the left knee. Wrap the left arm behind you and twist to the left, looking over the left shoulder as far as possible without strain. Hold this position breathing gently for about 10—15 seconds. Then relax, turn forward, and repeat the process, twisting to the right. Repeat 1—2 times in each direction.

We would like to give special thanks to one of the exercise models for this book: **Ethel Buerger,** age 71, Cleveland, Ohio

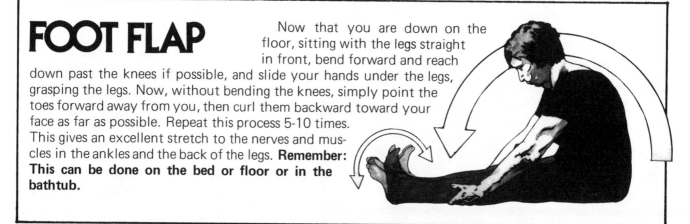

FOOT FLAP

Now that you are down on the floor, sitting with the legs straight in front, bend forward and reach down past the knees if possible, and slide your hands under the legs, grasping the legs. Now, without bending the knees, simply point the toes forward away from you, then curl them backward toward your face as far as possible. Repeat this process 5-10 times. This gives an excellent stretch to the nerves and muscles in the ankles and the back of the legs. **Remember: This can be done on the bed or floor or in the bathtub.**

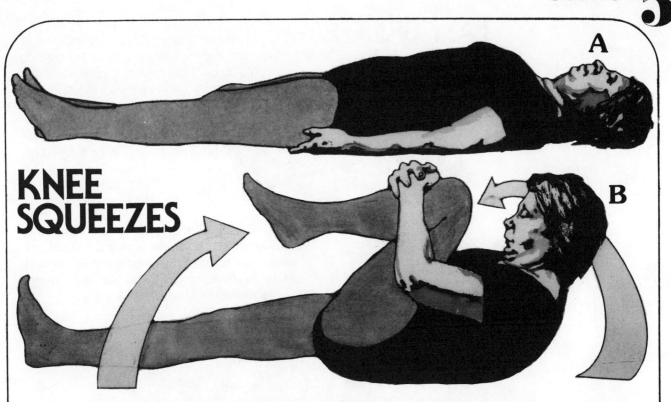

KNEE SQUEEZES

Lie flat on your back with your arms to your sides, palms up **(A).** Begin to breathe in as you raise the left knee to the chest **(B).** Fill your lungs about ½ to ¼ capacity and reach around the leg with your arms. Hold your breath as you squeeze the knee to the chest for 3-5 seconds. Exhale slowly as you straighten the leg and lower it slowly to the floor **(A).** Repeat process with opposite leg. Do 3 repetitions with each leg. When you get a little stronger, you can try to lift both legs and squeeze, as in Position **(C).** You can also raise your head toward the knee. **Remember: Move slowly and breathe through your nose smoothly. Do not strain. Hold the breath no longer than 5 seconds. Lower the legs and head slowly.**

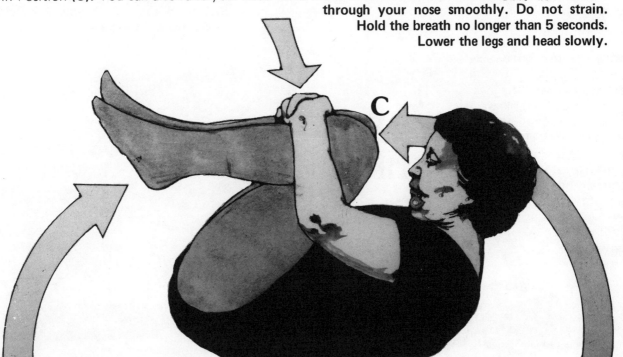

EASY BRIDGE

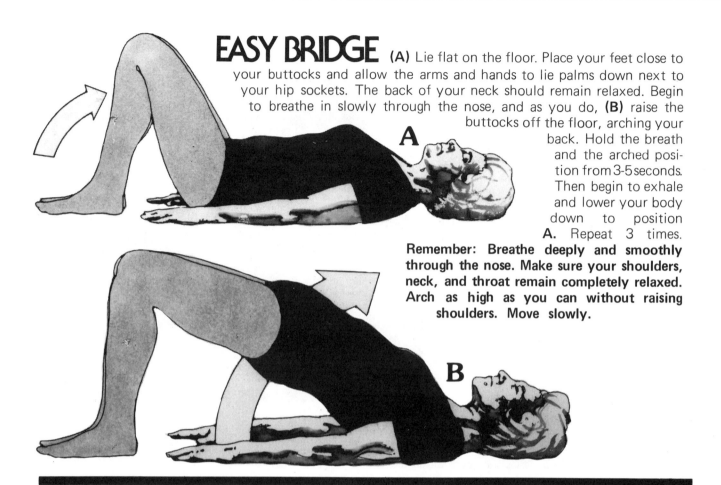

(A) Lie flat on the floor. Place your feet close to your buttocks and allow the arms and hands to lie palms down next to your hip sockets. The back of your neck should remain relaxed. Begin to breathe in slowly through the nose, and as you do, **(B)** raise the buttocks off the floor, arching your back. Hold the breath and the arched position from 3-5 seconds. Then begin to exhale and lower your body down to position A. Repeat 3 times.

Remember: Breathe deeply and smoothly through the nose. Make sure your shoulders, neck, and throat remain completely relaxed. Arch as high as you can without raising shoulders. Move slowly.

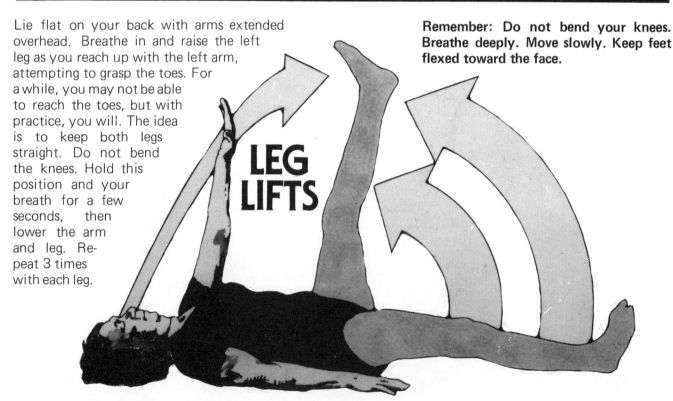

Lie flat on your back with arms extended overhead. Breathe in and raise the left leg as you reach up with the left arm, attempting to grasp the toes. For a while, you may not be able to reach the toes, but with practice, you will. The idea is to keep both legs straight. Do not bend the knees. Hold this position and your breath for a few seconds, then lower the arm and leg. Repeat 3 times with each leg.

LEG LIFTS

Remember: Do not bend your knees. Breathe deeply. Move slowly. Keep feet flexed toward the face.

54

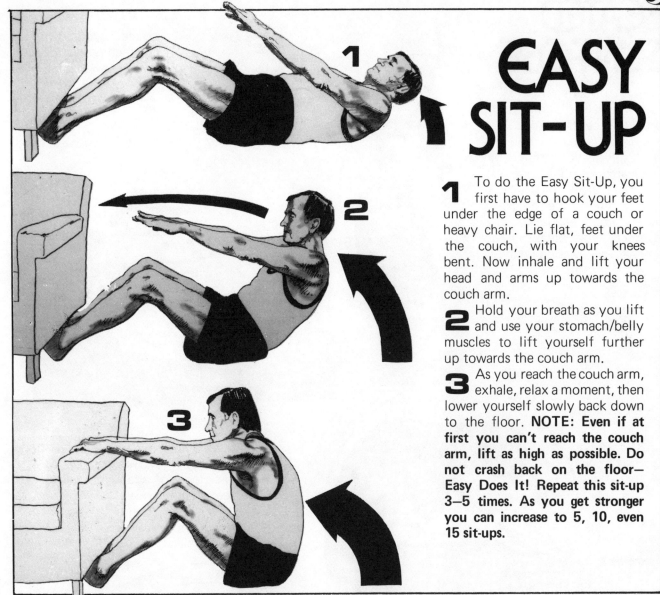

EASY SIT-UP

1 To do the Easy Sit-Up, you first have to hook your feet under the edge of a couch or heavy chair. Lie flat, feet under the couch, with your knees bent. Now inhale and lift your head and arms up towards the couch arm.

2 Hold your breath as you lift and use your stomach/belly muscles to lift yourself further up towards the couch arm.

3 As you reach the couch arm, exhale, relax a moment, then lower yourself slowly back down to the floor. **NOTE: Even if at first you can't reach the couch arm, lift as high as possible. Do not crash back on the floor—Easy Does It! Repeat this sit-up 3—5 times. As you get stronger you can increase to 5, 10, even 15 sit-ups.**

EASY FISH ARCH

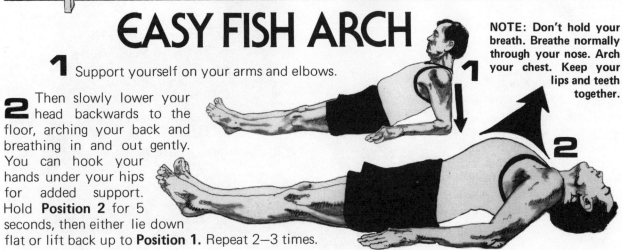

1 Support yourself on your arms and elbows.

2 Then slowly lower your head backwards to the floor, arching your back and breathing in and out gently. You can hook your hands under your hips for added support. Hold **Position 2** for 5 seconds, then either lie down flat or lift back up to **Position 1.** Repeat 2—3 times.

NOTE: Don't hold your breath. Breathe normally through your nose. Arch your chest. Keep your lips and teeth together.

55

SEATED SUN POSE

1 Sit up straight with your legs straight and your toes flexed back towards the face. Breathe in deeply as you stretch your arms to either side and raise them in a wide circle, filling the lungs. When your hands touch overhead, your lungs should be completely full.

2 Now slowly exhale as you bend forward. Lower the chin towards the chest and slowly dive towards the toes as you breathe out. Your lungs should be empty when you reach the legs.

3 Grasp as far down the legs as possible and wrap the hands underneath the knees, calves, or ankles. Your knees should remain straight. Do not strain; go only as far as is comfortable.

4 Bend the elbows to bring the chest down towards the thighs. Hold the breath out as you do so. Hold for 3—5 seconds. Now breathe in deeply and raise the arms up overhead as in **Position 1,** and then lower the arms down to your sides as you exhale. Repeat 3 times.

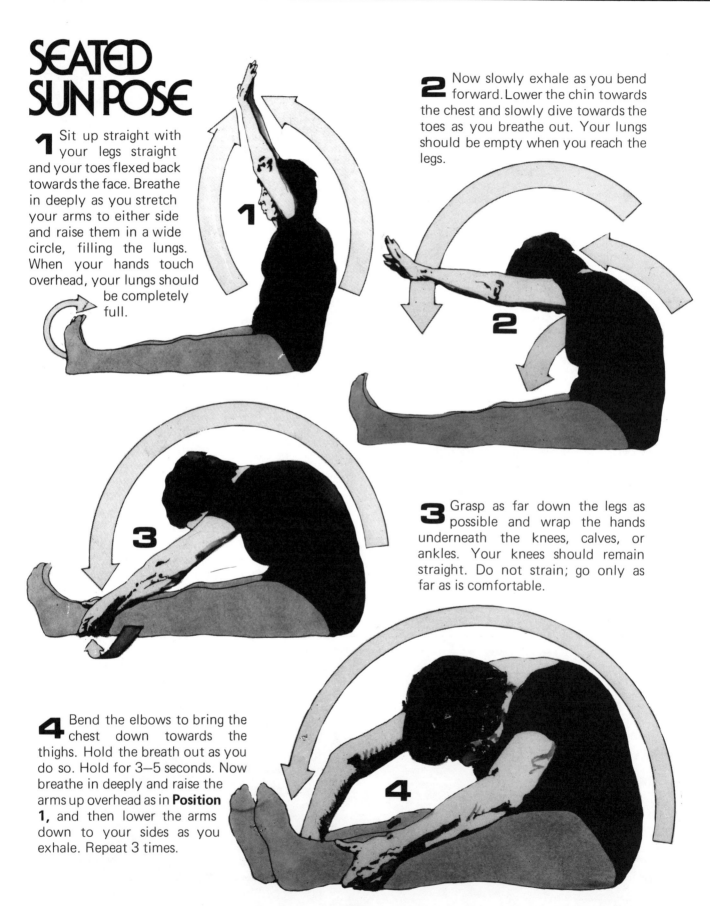

ALTERNATE SIDE STRETCH

1 This is essentially a side-to-side stretch for each leg and for your back. Sit up straight and spread your feet about 2—3 feet apart. Flex your feet backwards and keep them slightly flexed throughout this exercise.

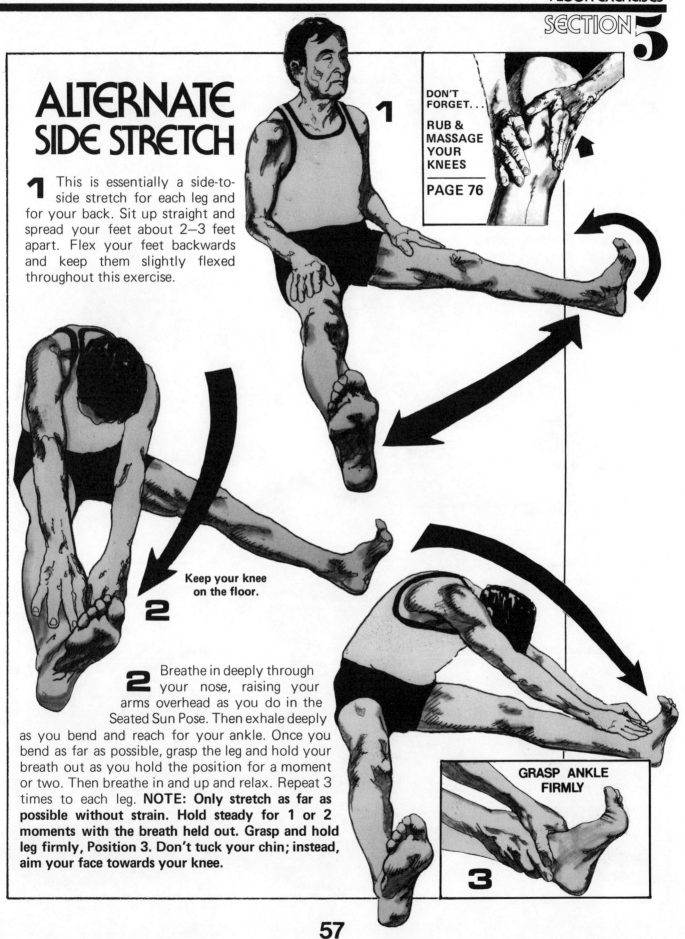

DON'T FORGET...
RUB & MASSAGE YOUR KNEES
PAGE 76

Keep your knee on the floor.

2 Breathe in deeply through your nose, raising your arms overhead as you do in the Seated Sun Pose. Then exhale deeply as you bend and reach for your ankle. Once you bend as far as possible, grasp the leg and hold your breath out as you hold the position for a moment or two. Then breathe in and up and relax. Repeat 3 times to each leg. **NOTE: Only stretch as far as possible without strain. Hold steady for 1 or 2 moments with the breath held out. Grasp and hold leg firmly, Position 3. Don't tuck your chin; instead, aim your face towards your knee.**

GRASP ANKLE FIRMLY

3

SPINE TWIST

Sit cross-legged on the floor. (A) Place your left hand on your right knee. Place your right hand behind you on the floor for support. Now twist to the right, looking backward over your right shoulder, as far as you can without straining. Hold this position (B) breathing gently for about 10 seconds; then relax. Turn forward and repeat in the opposite direction. Repeat process 2-3 times in each direction.

Remember: Breathe gently. Twist and move slowly. Keep your eyes open, staring at one spot on the wall behind you.

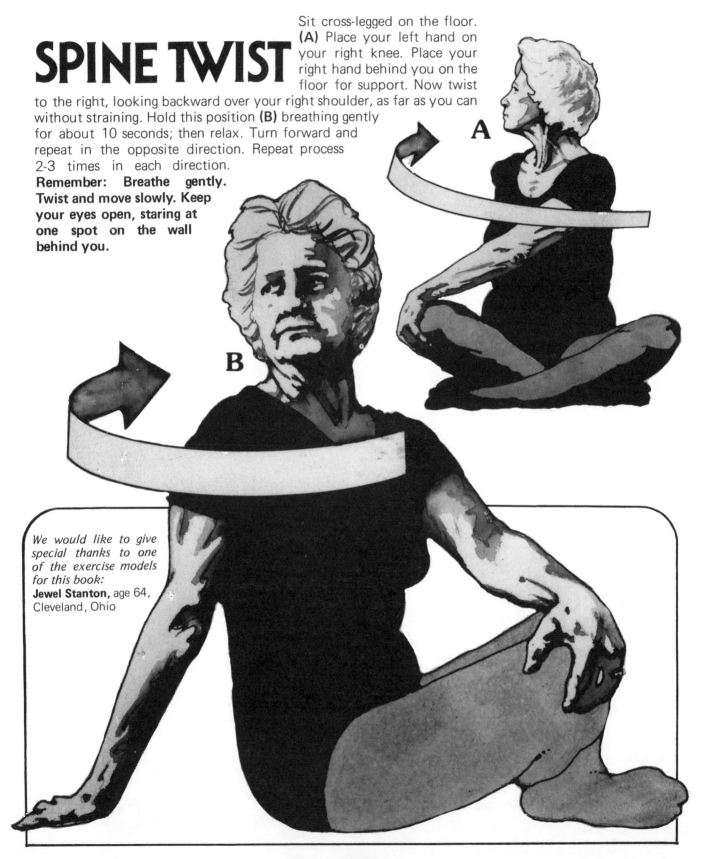

We would like to give special thanks to one of the exercise models for this book:
Jewel Stanton, age 64, Cleveland, Ohio

58

LOWER BACK STRETCH

This exercise gives a very nice stretch to the lower back and also the arms and upper chest.

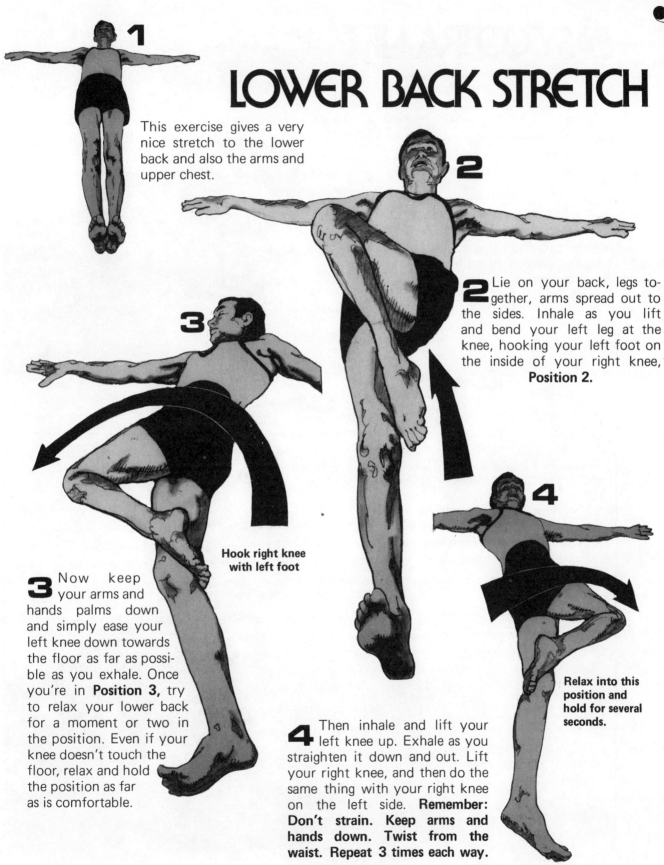

2 Lie on your back, legs together, arms spread out to the sides. Inhale as you lift and bend your left leg at the knee, hooking your left foot on the inside of your right knee, **Position 2.**

Hook right knee with left foot

3 Now keep your arms and hands palms down and simply ease your left knee down towards the floor as far as possible as you exhale. Once you're in **Position 3,** try to relax your lower back for a moment or two in the position. Even if your knee doesn't touch the floor, relax and hold the position as far as is comfortable.

Relax into this position and hold for several seconds.

4 Then inhale and lift your left knee up. Exhale as you straighten it down and out. Lift your right knee, and then do the same thing with your right knee on the left side. **Remember: Don't strain. Keep arms and hands down. Twist from the waist. Repeat 3 times each way.**

59

EASY COBRA LIFT

Lie down on your belly, then raise up so that you support yourself with your arms as in Position **(A)**. The arms should be perpendicular to the floor, forming a 90° right angle. They should not be angled out to the sides. Now as you breathe in gently, raise the head up and back as far as possible **(B)**. Hold this position for a few moments, breathing gently, lifting up with the back muscles. Then breathe out and lower the head toward the hands, stretching and relaxing the neck **(A)**.
Repeat 3 times.

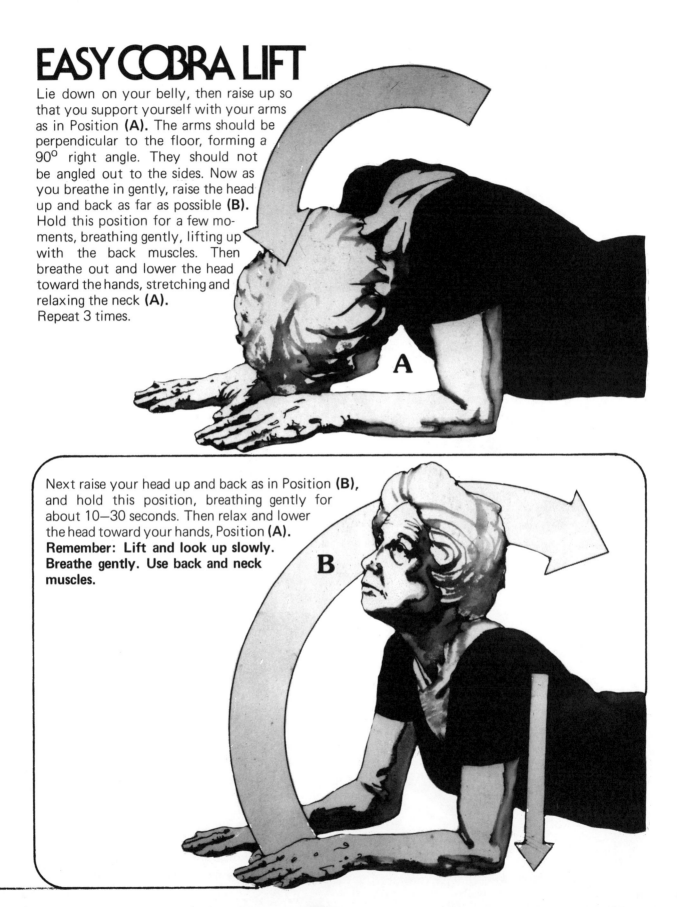

Next raise your head up and back as in Position **(B)**, and hold this position, breathing gently for about 10—30 seconds. Then relax and lower the head toward your hands, Position **(A)**.
Remember: Lift and look up slowly. Breathe gently. Use back and neck muscles.

60

COBRA TWIST

Lie down on your belly as you did in Position **(A)** of the Cobra Lift on the previous page. Slowly lift your head as you did in the Cobra Lift, but after reaching Position **(B)**, twist the head and neck and look to the extreme right. Then move the head very slowly to the extreme left. Go slowly back and forth 3 times.

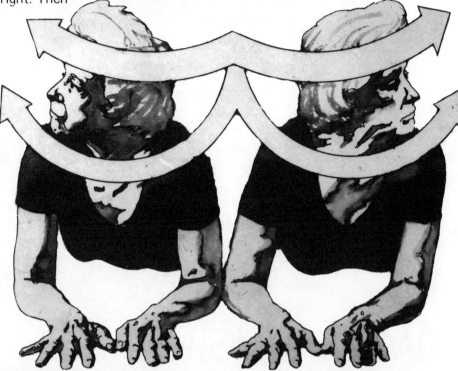

The Cobra Pose exercises are an excellent way to restore limberness and flexibility in the neck and shoulder areas. Many students report that because they practice the Cobra Poses every day, they are now able to turn their heads and look over their shoulders when driving a car or riding a bike.

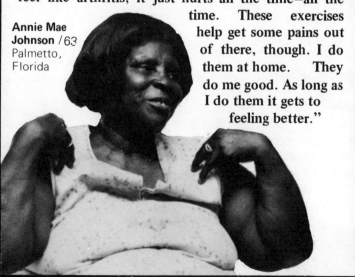

"Before this Yoga I didn't know nothing about rubbing and stretching and trying to get relief. Just moving them old bones I'd get to crying and crying I don't know what it is, one of the doctors says arthritis. It doesn't feel like arthritis, it just hurts all the time—all the time. These exercises help get some pains out of there, though. I do them at home. They do me good. As long as I do them it gets to feeling better."

Annie Mae Johnson / 63
Palmetto, Florida

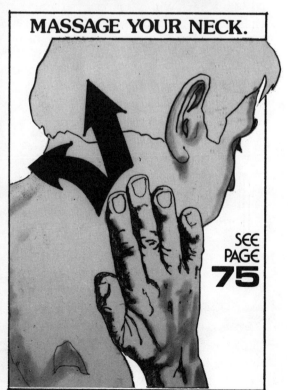

MASSAGE YOUR NECK.

SEE PAGE **75**

61

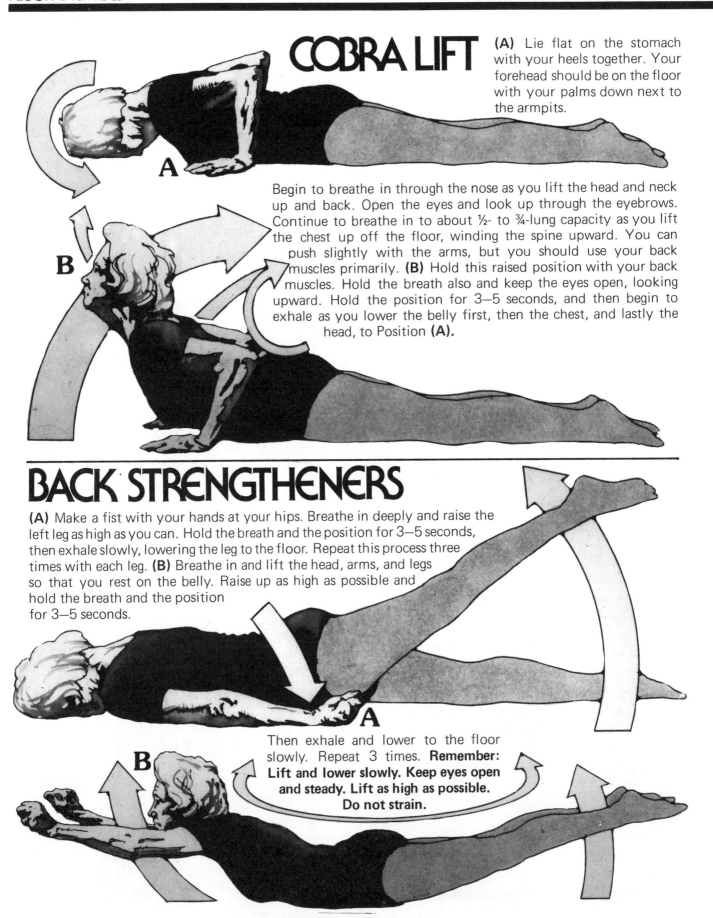

COBRA LIFT

(A) Lie flat on the stomach with your heels together. Your forehead should be on the floor with your palms down next to the armpits.

Begin to breathe in through the nose as you lift the head and neck up and back. Open the eyes and look up through the eyebrows. Continue to breathe in to about ½- to ¾-lung capacity as you lift the chest up off the floor, winding the spine upward. You can push slightly with the arms, but you should use your back muscles primarily. **(B)** Hold this raised position with your back muscles. Hold the breath also and keep the eyes open, looking upward. Hold the position for 3–5 seconds, and then begin to exhale as you lower the belly first, then the chest, and lastly the head, to Position **(A).**

BACK STRENGTHENERS

(A) Make a fist with your hands at your hips. Breathe in deeply and raise the left leg as high as you can. Hold the breath and the position for 3–5 seconds, then exhale slowly, lowering the leg to the floor. Repeat this process three times with each leg. **(B)** Breathe in and lift the head, arms, and legs so that you rest on the belly. Raise up as high as possible and hold the breath and the position for 3–5 seconds.

Then exhale and lower to the floor slowly. Repeat 3 times. **Remember: Lift and lower slowly. Keep eyes open and steady. Lift as high as possible. Do not strain.**

ALL FOURS LEG LIFTS

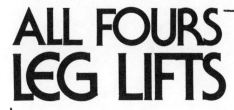

1 This exercise will help strengthen your lower back and legs. Breathe in deeply through your nose as you lift your right leg up and back as high as possible. Hold your breath and the position for a moment, and then exhale slowly as you lower your leg to the floor. **Repeat this exercise 3 times on each leg slowly and gently.**

2 Now study **Illustrations 2 & 3.** You will notice that in this variation you lift the right leg as you lift the left arm. Then you repeat it with the left leg and the right arm. **This not only strengthens the back muscles, but also the brain/nerve coordination that is so important to older people.**

In a variation of this exercise, which is not illustrated, you will raise the same arm as the leg. Watch your balance, because this is more difficult than the previous exercise. Breathe in slowly as you raise your **right** arm and **right** leg together. Then hold your breath and the position for a moment. Exhale slowly as you lower your arm and leg to the floor. **Repeat on each side 3 times. Hold the breath and position as steady as possible. Focus your eyes on the middle fingernail of the raised hand. Be sure to watch your balance.**

We would like to give special thanks to one of the exercise models for this book: **Robert Nelson,** age 62, Euclid, Ohio

SHOULDER STAND

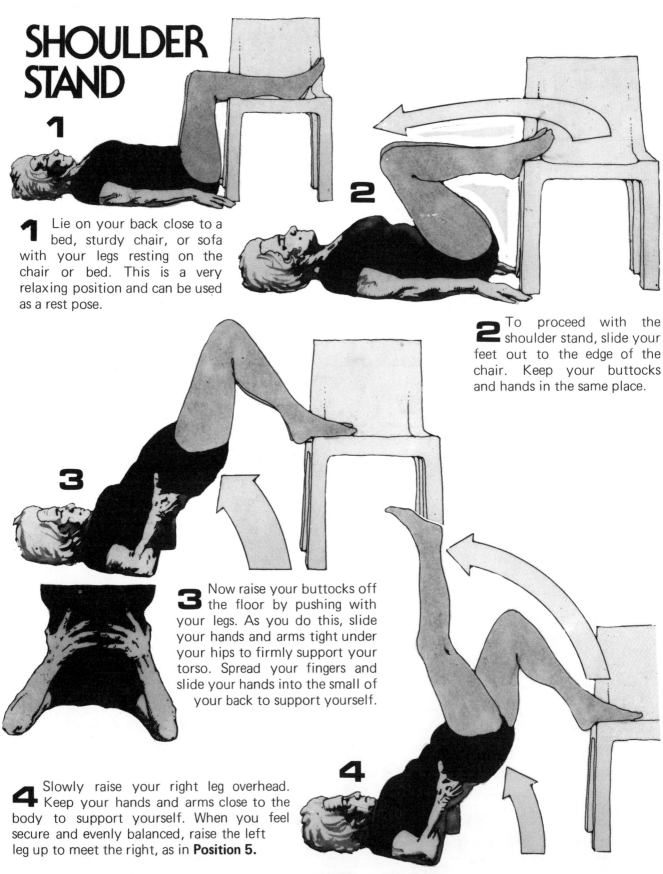

1

1 Lie on your back close to a bed, sturdy chair, or sofa with your legs resting on the chair or bed. This is a very relaxing position and can be used as a rest pose.

2

2 To proceed with the shoulder stand, slide your feet out to the edge of the chair. Keep your buttocks and hands in the same place.

3

3 Now raise your buttocks off the floor by pushing with your legs. As you do this, slide your hands and arms tight under your hips to firmly support your torso. Spread your fingers and slide your hands into the small of your back to support yourself.

4 Slowly raise your right leg overhead. Keep your hands and arms close to the body to support yourself. When you feel secure and evenly balanced, raise the left leg up to meet the right, as in **Position 5.**

4

INVERTED REST POSE

From **Position 5** lower both thighs to your chest while supporting your buttocks with your hands and arms. Relax the back of the neck and shoulders. Breathe gently and in a very relaxed manner with the eyes closed. Hold this position for 30 seconds, increasing to 2—3 minutes as you find it more comfortable. As you get more comfortable, you may also be able to rest your knees on your forehead or shoulders. To come out of this position, follow the same procedure as the shoulder stand. **Remember: Inverting the body like this may feel strange at first, but it is excellent for you. Move slowly. Breathe gently. Do not hold the breath.**

5 The legs and feet should be together and your shoulders should be relaxed. Hold the position and look at your toes with a steady, unblinking gaze. Breathe gently and relax in the position as much as you can. In the beginning you should hold the position for ten seconds, and over a period of weeks, gradually work up to about a minute.

TO DESCEND: Lower one foot to the edge of the chair. **Do not lower both legs at once,** as you might lose your balance. Proceed to **Position 3,** then **2,** and finally rest for a couple of minutes in **Position 1. Remember: throughout this exercise, move slowly —DO NOT HOLD the breath.** Breathe gently supporting the body with the arms and shoulders.

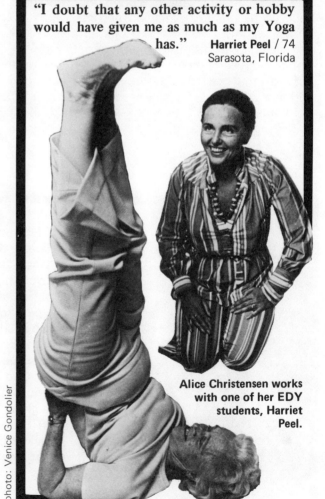

"I doubt that any other activity or hobby would have given me as much as my Yoga has." **Harriet Peel** / 74 Sarasota, Florida

Alice Christensen works with one of her EDY students, Harriet Peel.

photo: Venice Gondolier

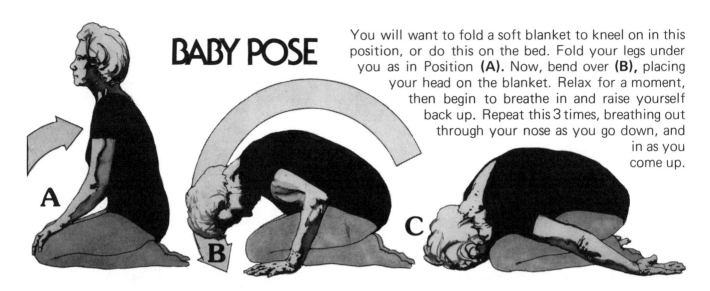

BABY POSE

You will want to fold a soft blanket to kneel on in this position, or do this on the bed. Fold your legs under you as in Position **(A)**. Now, bend over **(B)**, placing your head on the blanket. Relax for a moment, then begin to breathe in and raise yourself back up. Repeat this 3 times, breathing out through your nose as you go down, and in as you come up.

Remember: Breathe deeply and move slowly. Relax. Next, simply fold in half, letting your arms hang to the sides. Rest your head on your blanket in front of the knees **(C)**. After you have done this for a few weeks, you will be able to hold the folded position more comfortably and will find it very enjoyable. Then relax your breathing and all of the tension in your shoulders, neck, and back. With practice, this will become very relaxing and refreshing. After you practice this for a few weeks, you can even nap in this position with excellent results. A similar exercise is shown in Position **(D)**. Lie on the edge of the bed so that the edge crosses your abdomen. Relax arms and head on the floor and hold this position, breathing gently, for 30 seconds to 3-5 minutes, depending on the ease of the position.

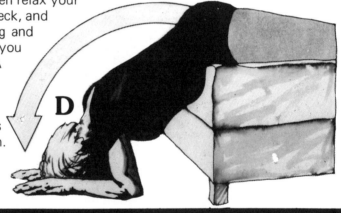

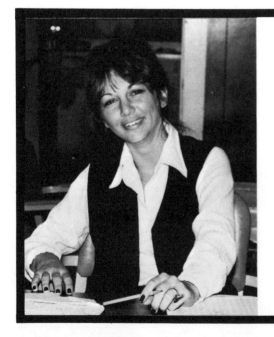

"It's really incredible. It was very apathetic around here before this *Easy Does It Yoga.* Older people have a tendency, when they are withdrawn and isolated, to just sort of hunch over and slump around. When they feel good about themselves and their bodies you can actually see it. They're just, you know, visibly different. They straighten up, they have a glow, and they're more outgoing! The people here really got into this Yoga. It really brought them out; now they talk to everybody about it. They're proud of themselves and what they've achieved. A lot of them are doing it at home, and you can really tell. They're just more energetic. They have a glow. They can stand up more, and they take more pride in themselves. They weren't into arts and crafts, or into field trips, or anything like that, but this Yoga, they really got into it!"

Dale Robbins, Site Director of Seffner Civic Center, Senior Citizen Nutrition & Activity Program, Seffner, Florida

SPECIAL EXERCISES SECTION 6

"In contrast to the Ohio Commission on Aging's physical fitness training sessions, The Light of Yoga Society proposed a series of sessions designed for the more frail elderly. Alice Christensen and David Rankin, two experts in the field, have designed a Yoga routine that can be done by persons who are confined to wheelchairs or who are even bedridden. The exercises help to promote flexibility and strength which are so important to those with arthritis or other musculoskeletal limitations. The program is a smashing success!"

SUSIE LENNOX-RIVERS, Executive Director,
Cuyahoga Area Agency on Aging, Cleveland, Ohio

IN THE BED

Of all the exercises in this book, the bed exercises are the most loved. Many older people suffer from severe morning stiffness or are incapable of getting down on the floor, some are convalescing, and others just like to exercise in bed. Whatever your situation, these exercises will help you get going in the morning and keep going all day. **In order to use this section, please note the page numbers of the exercises you want to do. Open to that page and do the exercise. After a while, you'll have a nice morning routine you can do easily.**

LOWER BACK STRETCH

SEE PAGE **59**

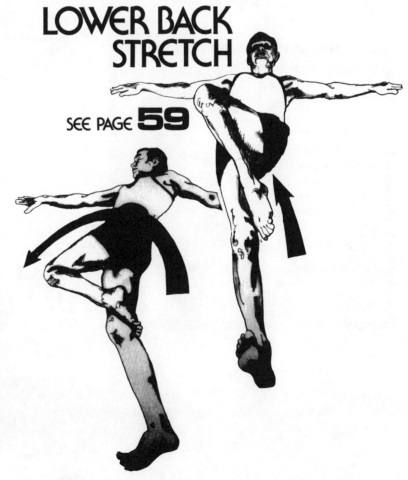

IN THE BED

KNEE SQUEEZES

SEE PAGE **53**

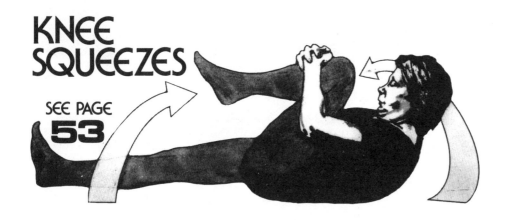

EASY BRIDGE

SEE PAGE **54**

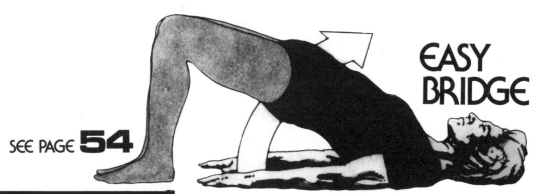

"I was in the hospital a year ago for some back trouble so I couldn't do some of the floor exercises. So I do a lot of those bed exercises and I always do these knee squeezes every morning before getting out of bed."

Pauline Moody
73
Bradenton, Florida

LEG LIFTS
SEE PAGE **54**

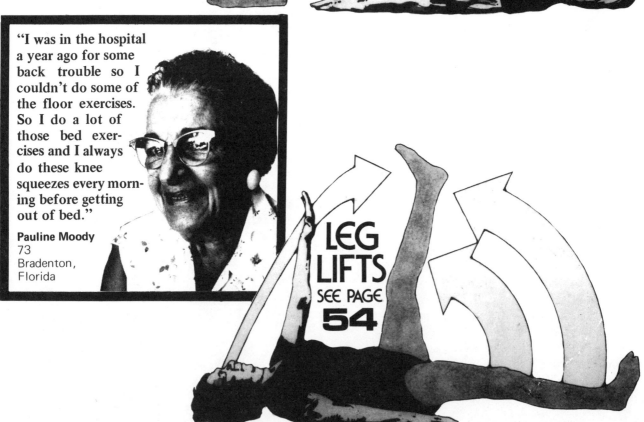

EASY FISH ARCH

SEE PAGE **55**

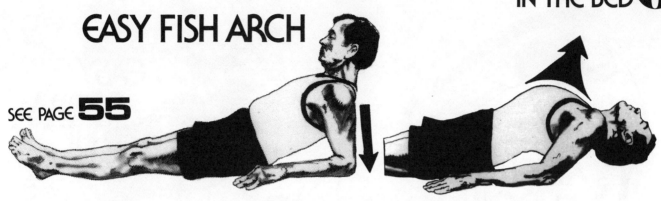

SEE PAGE **52**
FOOT FLAP

GENTLE TWIST

SEE PAGE **52**

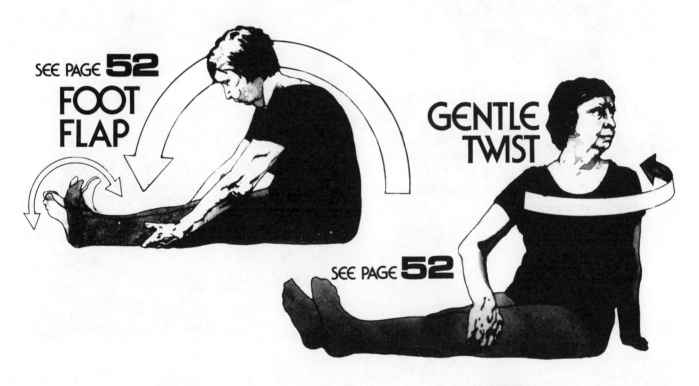

EASY SIT-UP
SEE PAGE **55**

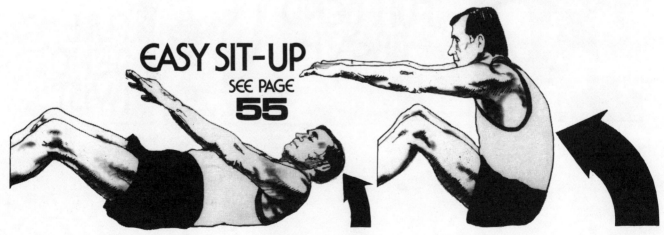

IN THE BED

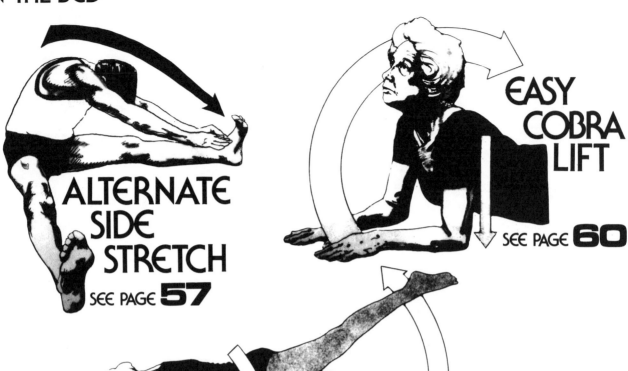

ALTERNATE SIDE STRETCH

SEE PAGE **57**

EASY COBRA LIFT

SEE PAGE **60**

BACK STRENGTHENERS

SEE PAGE **62**

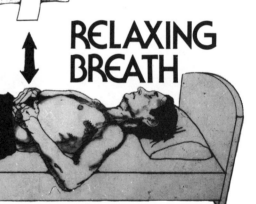

RELAXING BREATH

SEE PAGE **86**

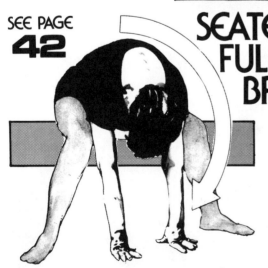

SEE PAGE **42**

SEATED FULL BEND BREATH

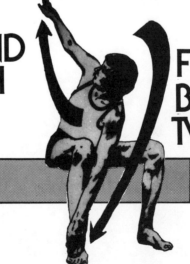

FULL BEND TWIST

SEE PAGE **42**

70

IN A WHEELCHAIR

Many people with severe disabilities have been able to help themselves by utilizing Easy Does It Yoga's simple approach. Even if you or a loved one is bedridden or confined to a wheelchair, chances are you can do at least a few of these Easy Does It Yoga exercises, especially the breathing and meditation.

"I'm a double amputee, and I get tired of just sitting around doing nothing. I really look forward to my Easy Does It Yoga. I practice at least four to five days a week and it makes me feel good. The breathing, relaxation, and exercises make me feel stronger and useful, and it's very nice. I enjoy it a lot!"

Buster Henderson
47
Palmetto, Florida

ARM ROTATIONS   SEE PAGE 38

HEAD ROTATIONS   SEE PAGE 36

ARM REACHES   SEE PAGE 37

SHOULDER SHRUGS   SEE PAGE 33

Begin with simple arm and shoulder exercises and work up to the more challenging ones as you get stronger and more confident. **Remember: Apply your brake before exercising so that your chair doesn't move as you bend and twist. Also, if possible, do the exercises on the opposite page with your feet on the floor, not on your chair's foot supports.**

LEG LIFTS

SEE PAGE 41

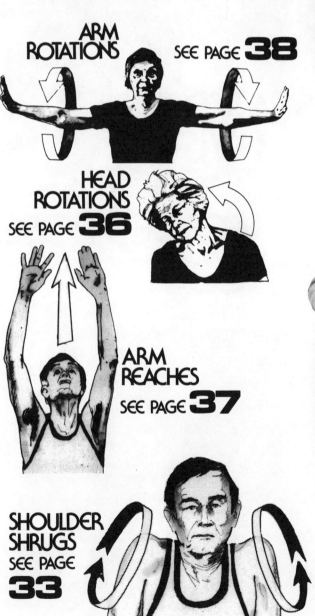

71

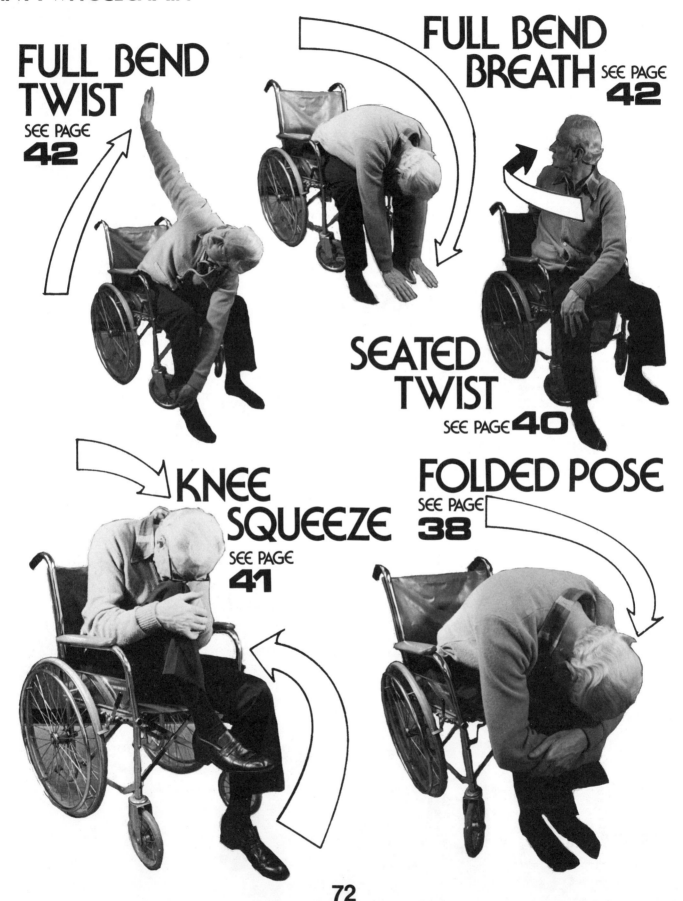

FULL BEND TWIST
SEE PAGE **42**

FULL BEND BREATH
SEE PAGE **42**

SEATED TWIST
SEE PAGE **40**

KNEE SQUEEZE
SEE PAGE **41**

FOLDED POSE
SEE PAGE **38**

DO THE FOLLOWING EVERY DAY:

BREATHING EXERCISES

HUMMING BREATH, COMPLETE BREATH, RELAXING BREATH, AND BELLY BREATH

SEE PAGES **83-86**

YOUR COMPLETE RELAXATION

A GRADUAL & SYSTEMATIC WAY TO RELEASE TENSIONS & GET COMPLETE REST.

SEE PAGES **89-90**

OM MEDITATION TECHNIQUE

THE MEDITATIVE ABILITY TO FOCUS AND RELAX THE MIND WITH THE SOUND OM.

SEE PAGES **91-92**

SAT-SILENT AWARENESS TRAINING

THE ABILITY TO EXTEND MEDITATIVE AWARENESS INTO PURE MENTAL SILENCE.

SEE PAGES **92-93**

EYE EXERCISE

EYE ROTATIONS

For most people, vision is the most important sense. Keeping the eye muscles toned and healthy is a primary ingredient of good vision as we get older. The following eye exercises can be done anytime and will be helpful in maintaining healthy eyes.

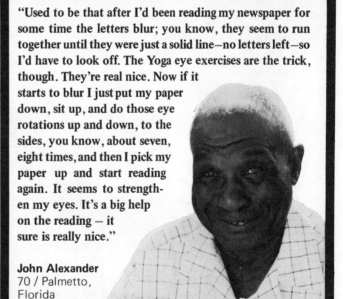

"Used to be that after I'd been reading my newspaper for some time the letters blur; you know, they seem to run together until they were just a solid line—no letters left—so I'd have to look off. The Yoga eye exercises are the trick, though. They're real nice. Now if it starts to blur I just put my paper down, sit up, and do those eye rotations up and down, to the sides, you know, about seven, eight times, and then I pick my paper up and start reading again. It seems to strengthen my eyes. It's a big help on the reading — it sure is really nice."

John Alexander
70 / Palmetto, Florida

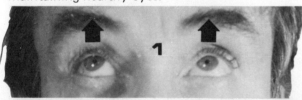

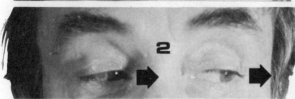

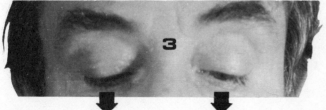

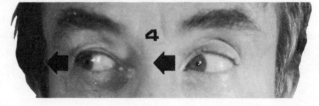

1. Open eyes wide and look up through your eyebrows. **2.** Then roll them down to the left. **3.** Continue and roll them straight down, **4.** and then up and over to the right. **Roll your eyes 3—5 rotations to the left, then 3—5 rotations to the right. As your eyes get stronger, increase rotations to 5—10 each way. Don't strain.**

FOCUSING

The Eye Rotations exercise the muscles that move the eyes up, down, and sideways. This exercise works on the muscles that focus vision within your eyes. Hold a pen, or even your thumb, out in front of you at arm's length, and stare at the tip of the pen until it is clearly focused in your vision. Then simply look away to the furthest point in your room, and focus your vision on a lamp or picture on the wall. After your eyes focus on the distant object, refocus them on the tip of the pencil again. You may feel the muscles of your eyes strain a little at first so only try a couple of times in the beginning. After a few days' practice you will be able to shift your focus from the tip of the pencil to the wall and back to the pencil 5, 10, 15 times in 30 seconds. The eyes may tear a little, but don't strain. **Begin with just a few wall-to-pencil focuses and build up slowly over the course of a week or two. Don't overdo; remember, this is exercise—so Easy Does It!**

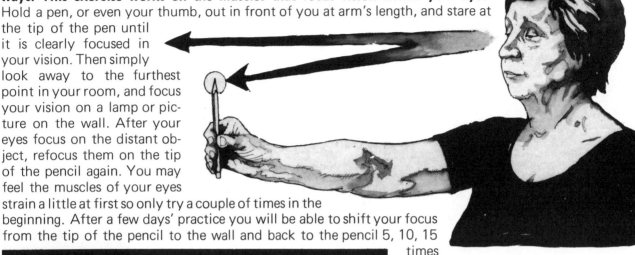

"I also do those eye exercises. If I don't have a pencil handy, I use my thumb. They have really helped my tired eyes."

Mae Norris
84
Bradenton,
Florida

EYE PALMING

This Yoga technique releases tension in the eyes after eye exercises, reading, TV, or any time your eyes are tired or strained. Press in gently on the eyes with the palms of your hands for 10—30 seconds. Then release pressure, wait a few moments, and repeat. Don't press too hard. **NOTE: This simple Yoga technique releases eye tension so that afterwards your vision may be blurred a few moments until your eyes re-tense and focus again. This is very healthy for your eyes and can even help relieve headaches.**

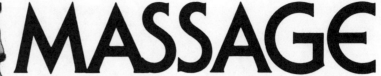

MASSAGE

Massaging your joints and muscles daily helps remove stiffness and aches and pains and helps circulation. It helps to incorporate these massage hints into your exercise routine as well as at various other times of your day—such as while you watch TV. **NOTE: Before massaging any part of your body, rub your hands together briskly until they feel warm with energy. This really helps.**

SHOULDERS—Rub the entire shoulder area with a firm, circular motion.

HEAD—Start from the temples and rub into the center and back out again. Do between your eyebrows and all the way up into your scalp.

NECK—Rub up and down from your throat all the way up and around the back of your neck. Rub firmly with fingers.

ELBOWS—Grasp your elbow joint firmly and rotate your hand back and forth around the entire elbow joint.

LOWER BACK—Place your hands firmly on your lower back and rub up and down all the way to your tail bone.

SHOULDERS

HEAD

NECK

ELBOWS

LOWER BACK

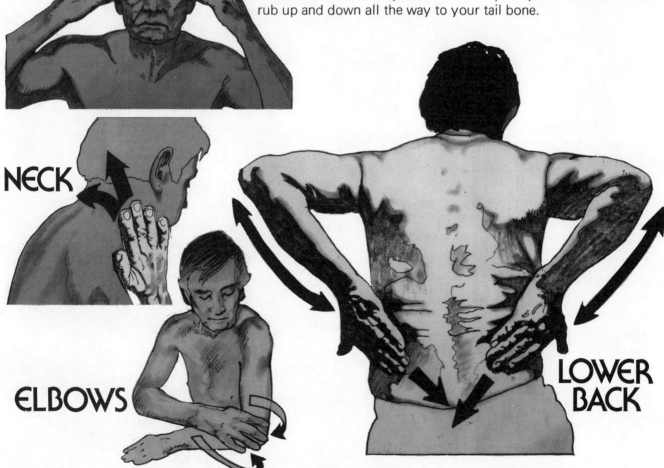

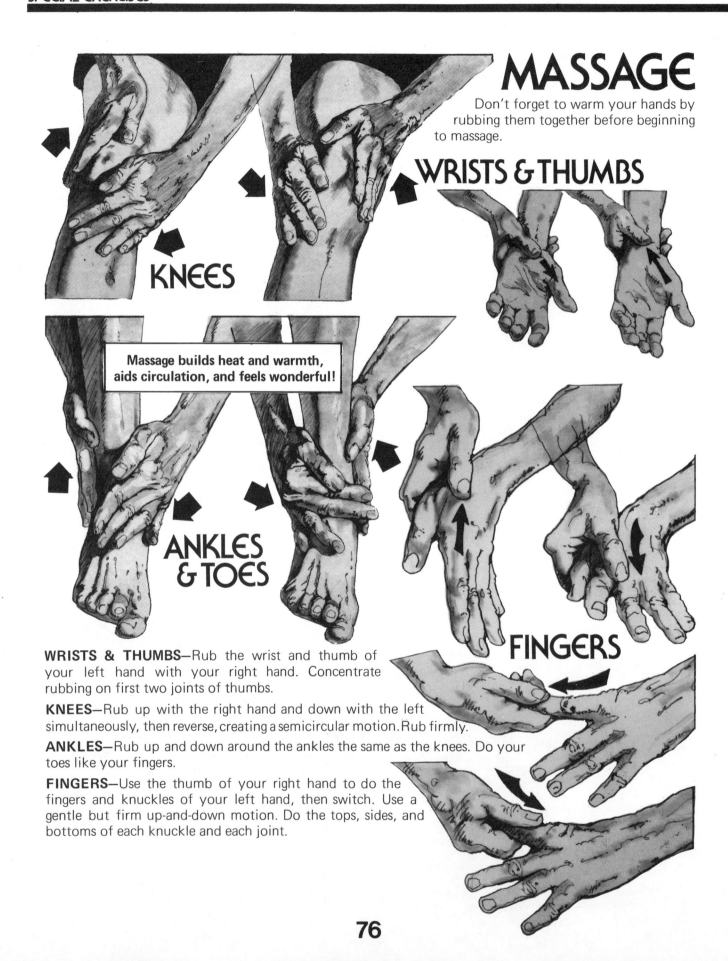

MASSAGE

Don't forget to warm your hands by rubbing them together before beginning to massage.

WRISTS & THUMBS

KNEES

Massage builds heat and warmth, aids circulation, and feels wonderful!

ANKLES & TOES

FINGERS

WRISTS & THUMBS—Rub the wrist and thumb of your left hand with your right hand. Concentrate rubbing on first two joints of thumbs.

KNEES—Rub up with the right hand and down with the left simultaneously, then reverse, creating a semicircular motion. Rub firmly.

ANKLES—Rub up and down around the ankles the same as the knees. Do your toes like your fingers.

FINGERS—Use the thumb of your right hand to do the fingers and knuckles of your left hand, then switch. Use a gentle but firm up-and-down motion. Do the tops, sides, and bottoms of each knuckle and each joint.

IN THE TUB

The warm water in your bath can help to limber you up and provide a safe environment for some simple exercises. Next time you're in your bath, try these few stretches and give your lower back, legs, and shoulders a massage in the hot water. **You'll not only be clean, but limber too!**

"The massaging is so nice—you can do it anytime—sometimes before my exercise, sometimes after, even in front of the TV. I even do it in the bathtub. It gets so nice and warm, and it really feels so good!"

Jeanne Hrovat
66
Euclid, Ohio

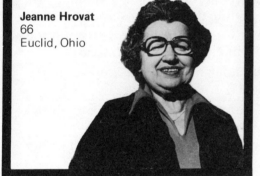

FOOT FLAP
SEE PAGE **52**

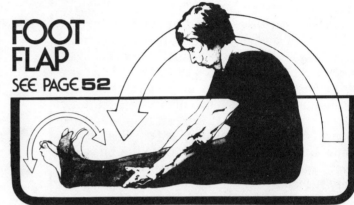

SEATED SUN POSE

SEE PAGE **56**

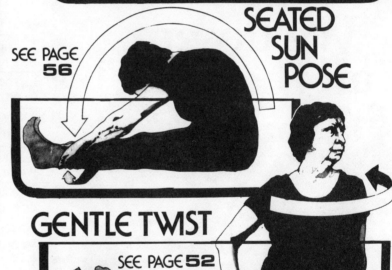

GENTLE TWIST

SEE PAGE **52**

TUB REACH

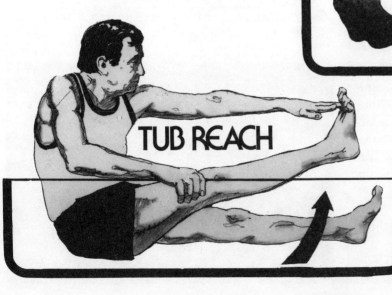

Straighten your legs and flex your toes back towards your face. Now grab the edge of the tub for support. Breathe through the nose as you raise your leg as high out of the water as you can. **Keep your knees straight.** Reach towards your feet and try to touch your toes. Hold the position and your breath for a moment and then exhale and slowly lower your leg. **Repeat three times on each leg.**

ANYTIME EXERCISES

One of the major aims of Easy Does It Yoga is to provide an easily applied fitness program that activates all areas of the body, breath, and mind. In this way it allows individuals to do the exercises and procedures throughout their daily lives, accommodating them to their individual needs, limitations and schedules. In this respect, Easy Does It Yoga is most successful in activating one's entire being, building self-confidence and total fitness. **The idea is to do a little bit wherever you are whenever you can. This results in easy success!**

"We do 'em all the time."

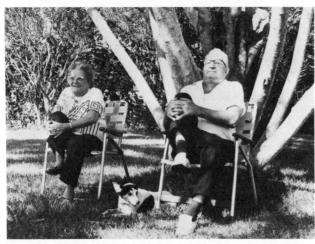

- "I do my foot flaps waiting for the bus."
- "I like to do my silent meditation in church."
- "When I'm waiting for the tea kettle to boil, I do the leg lifts."
- "The eye palming relaxes my eyes during TV commercials."
- "Talking on the phone is a great opportunity to do my leg lifts."
- "Waiting in the dentist's office, the Yoga breathing helps me relax."
- "Now I practice getting up and down off the floor while I watch TV."
- "I do those twisting poses in the car at stoplights."
- "That complete relaxation procedure is great in the late afternoon instead of a nap."
- "I improve my balance by standing on one leg while doing the dishes."
- "In the grocery store line I do my tip toe breath while holding onto the cart."
- "The shoulder massage is a lifesaver in the morning."
- "I do elbow rolls and shoulder shrugs when I brush my teeth."
- "The bed exercises are the way I start my day, every day."
- "Now we take a short exercise break between hands of bridge."
- "When I'm on my bike I love to do my deep breathing exercises."
- "I relax and do my meditation after the soaps in the afternoon."

"Whenever I'm just sitting I try to do some Yoga—I never waste time just sitting watching TV. Instead of just sitting there all slouched over, I do leg lifts, knee squeezes, and the bending over ones. I do my foot flaps and breathing and twisting. It limbers you up while you watch TV. And you know, after exercising, you feel better instead of all tired. You feel like getting up and doing something or going out.

Jeanne Hrovat / 66 / Euclid, Ohio

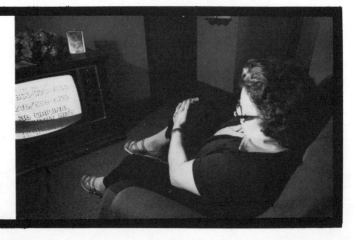

BREATHING EXERCISES 7

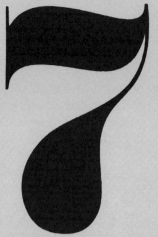

SECTION

YOU FILL YOUR STOMACH WITH 3 MEALS A DAY, BUT
YOU FILL YOUR LUNGS WITH AIR
30,000 TIMES A DAY!

BREATH IS YOUR MOST PRECIOUS POSSESSION.

There is nothing in your life more important to you than the air you breathe. People have been known to go for weeks without food and for days without water. However, if you breathe all the air out of your lungs and try to finish reading just this one page, you won't make it.

Your lungs have been in continuous motion since the day you were born. The average 70-year-old person breathes 2,300 gallons of air each day, but despite the vital importance of breath to every aspect of our lives and the massive quantities of air we move each day, most of us never think about our breathing.

The amount of air you breathe in your lifetime would fill over 50 Goodyear Blimps.

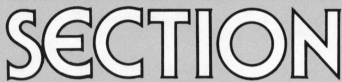

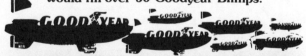

"I got more pep, more energy. A lot more energy! There were times when I could hardly finish my lunch. I'd have to lay down and take a nap. I still take naps once in a while, but I don't need them like I used to. And I think it's the breathing exercises that's done that!"

Josephine Vidmar, 70
Cleveland, Ohio

People who practice Yoga learn not to take their breath for granted. For thousands of years, Yoga has taught people how to train the breath in order to lengthen life and improve physical/mental health. An ancient book on Yoga, the *Aitareya Upanishad,* written in 300 B.C., states: *"The breath forms the foundation on which the whole base of the body and mind rest."*

POOR BREATHING ROBS YOU OF ENERGY & LIFE.

Normal aging processes will rob you of thirty to forty gallons of air each hour unless you learn to breathe better. In one day, at age 70, you get nine gallons less pure oxygen in your blood than at age 30, if you let age take its course. You were breathing 135 gallons of air per hour, and now you are breathing only 95 gallons per hour. This decreased breathing causes a 20-25% reduction in the amount of oxygen you have in your blood. Poor breathing is literally robbing you of energy and life.

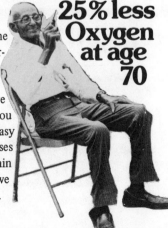

25% less Oxygen at age 70

If you could regain the oxygen and energy lost in just one day, it would be enough energy to allow you to walk two miles briskly or play cards for 2½ hours. You could do more of the things that you like if you had more energy. Your Easy Does It Yoga breathing exercises help you to immediately regain some of this lost energy and live a longer, fuller, healthier life.

►YOU MAY BE SUFFERING FROM SLOW SUFFOCATION.◄

Unless you exercise your breathing, aging affects the respiratory system in the following three areas:

STIFFNESS Breathing in becomes more difficult because the rib cage and surrounding muscles get stiffer as we get older. These muscles normally expand the chest when breathing in, helping the diaphragm draw in air. When breathing out, the muscles squeeze the rib cage, helping to force air out of the lungs. Breathing muscles must be gently stretched and strengthened, and the joints of the ribs at the breastbone and spine must be limbered to restore easy breathing. Your EDY will help you do this.

LOST ELASTICITY & WEAK MUSCLES As you age, the lungs gradually lose their elasticity, and consequently, their ability to return to their original size as we breathe out. This means that stale air remains in the lung tissues and must be forced out by the muscles in the chest and belly. However, these muscles weaken with age, making it difficult to empty the lungs completely. When you start to breathe in again, the stale air still in the tissues of the lungs prevents fresh oxygen from reaching the bloodstream. Your EDY breathing exercises will strengthen weakened breathing muscles and make your lung tissues elastic and healthy again.

RAPID, SHALLOW BREATHING Poor posture, stiffness, weak muscles, and loss of lung tissue elasticity collectively contribute to a rapid, shallow breathing pattern in most older people. This in turn results in poor oxygen supply, respiratory disease, sluggishness, senility, and heart disease. Rapid, shallow breathers move air in and out of just the upper portion of the lungs, while the lower lung regions contain stale air. Gravity, however, pulls most of the blood supply to the lower lungs. This means that the fresh, oxygen-rich air in the upper lungs does not reach the lower lungs and bloodstream. Hence, this inefficient breathing pattern lowers the oxygen level of the body and brain. Lying down, then, makes breathing even more inefficient, and oxygen levels may fall so low during sleep that many older people suffer from nighttime confusion, loss of memory, and severe disorientation. EDY breathing exercises

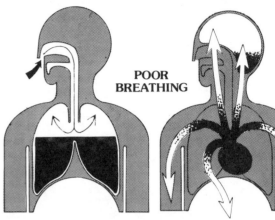

Poor breathing allows the lower lung space to go unused.

This results in poor oxygen supply to the blood, brain, and body.

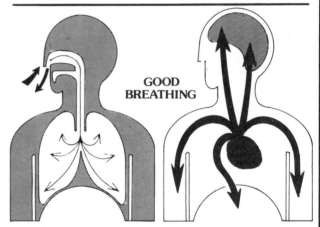

EDY breathing exercises help you to utilize your fullest lung capacity. This full lung usage results in better oxygenation of the blood, reduced breath and heart rate, and improved overall health and energy.

will help you get more oxygen deeper into the lower lungs and reduce your respiration rate, thereby reducing strain on your heart.

QUIT SMOKING
SMOKING IS THE MAJOR CAUSE OF:

**CANCER
HEART DISEASE
EMPHYSEMA
BRONCHITIS**

If you add smoking to the normal breathing difficulties associated with aging, you have an even more difficult problem. If you use tobacco you already know the shortness of breath, the chronic cough, and the painful, tiring breathing you suffer with. You also probably know someone who is dying of emphysema, lung cancer, or other smoking-related illness. Why do you continue with each cigarette to bring yourself closer to the horror of such a slow and painful death?

ARE YOU A SLOUCH?

As people settle into a life style of greater inactivity they develop a tendency to sit more and more. The more you sit, the weaker you become. How you hold your body indicates how you feel about yourself and your life. The Slouch can become the body position of chronic inactivity. It is also a physical position indicative of depression, fatigue, sluggishness, feelings of loss, and despondency.

The first step toward better breathing and renewed energy is to determine whether or not you're a slouch. If you sit in The Slouch Position for more than 1½ hours per day without some major movement of the body, then you're a slouch. This doesn't mean that you should never relax or settle into a comfortable chair to read or watch TV. However, unless you get some exercise, even in your chair, The Slouch Position can become extremely debilitating.

It should be understood that prolonged time spent in The Slouch Position:

1. weakens all postural muscles in the back;
2. weakens all abdominal muscles;
3. systematically reduces oxygen to the body and brain;
4. upsets vital functioning of the intestines, bladder, kidneys, and prostate;
5. weakens the hip sockets, lower back, and neck;
6. weakens the legs;
7. decreases energy levels;
8. cuts off blood circulation.

Oddly enough, people think this is resting, yet prolonged sitting in The Slouch actually weakens the heart and arteries and contributes to strokes.

● WHAT YOU CAN DO ABOUT THE SLOUCH...

1. DO THE CHAIR EXERCISES IN SECTION 3 WHILE YOU WATCH TV SO THAT YOU REMAIN ACTIVE EVEN WHILE YOU SIT.
2. DO THE STANDING AND FLOOR EXERCISES IN SECTIONS 4 and 5; THESE WILL IMPROVE YOUR POSTURAL MUSCLES AND BLOOD CIRCULATION.
3. DO THE BREATHING EXERCISES ON THE FOLLOWING PAGES.

OVERWEIGHT?

Due to inactivity, illness and poor eating habits, many older people suffer from chronic overweight problems. Carrying so much weight around your mid-section represents a major contributing factor in breathing abnormalities, heart problems, and spinal injury.

Breathing Exercise helps reduce heart, lung, & spinal strain.

Excess weight weakens the abdominal muscles causing a tremendous downward pull on the heart and lungs. This downward pull makes the lungs work inefficiently as they can neither expel stale air effectively nor can they get fresh oxygen rich air deep enough into the lungs. Your heart is also forced to work extra hard in order to compensate.

HEART AND LUNGS

Your spine and muscles support your entire upper body weight. Excess weight strains the shoulder and neck muscles and can cause slippage of the vertebrae and spinal discs.

Excess weight also weakens and strains the lower back and pulls the spine forward dramatically. This can cause severe lower back pain, slippage of discs and vertebrae and even spinal injury and paralysis.

It is our hope that through your EDY you will begin to lose weight and keep it off, allowing you to live longer and healthier. The breathing exercises on the following pages will help strengthen weak abdominal muscles and lessen heart strain.

HOW DOES BREATHING WORK?

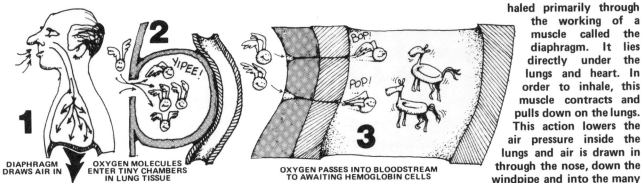

1 DIAPHRAGM DRAWS AIR IN

OXYGEN MOLECULES ENTER TINY CHAMBERS IN LUNG TISSUE

3 OXYGEN PASSES INTO BLOODSTREAM TO AWAITING HEMOGLOBIN CELLS

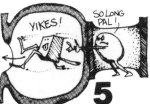

4 HEMOGLOBIN CELLS CARRY OXYGEN ALL OVER THE BODY

5 THE BLOODSTREAM CARRIES CARBON DIOXIDE BACK TO THE TINY LUNG CHAMBERS

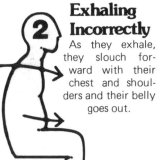

6 FROM THERE CARBON DIOXIDE PASSES INTO LUNGS

7 AND FINALLY IS EXHALED OUT OF THE BODY

■**1** Air is inhaled and exhaled primarily through the working of a muscle called the diaphragm. It lies directly under the lungs and heart. In order to inhale, this muscle contracts and pulls down on the lungs. This action lowers the air pressure inside the lungs and air is drawn in through the nose, down the windpipe and into the many tree-like branches of the lungs. ■**2** The air you breathe is approximately 21% oxygen, and the main objective of inhalation is to get these oxygen molecules deep down into millions of tiny chambers in the lung tissues, called alveoli. ■**3** These tiny chambers are surrounded by tiny blood vessels (capillaries). The marvelous thing is that the oxygen molecules pass right through the thin membranes of the lungs and blood vessels to the waiting blood cells called hemoglobin. ■**4** Once in the bloodstream, the hemoglobin carries the oxygen all over the body, where it is used in cell metabolism to allow us to do all the things we do.

■**5** As we move about, and even during rest, another gaseous molecule, called carbon dioxide, is produced as a waste product that is picked up by the bloodstream, returned to the lungs, and pushed out into the tiny lung chambers. ■**6** These carbon dioxide molecules are further expelled back into the lungs and... ■**7** Then the diaphragm muscle relaxes, the lungs decrease in size, which increases the internal air pressure, forcing the air out of the chest in what we commonly call exhaling. Thus, in this process, vital, life-giving oxygen is drawn into the body and the unusable waste product carbon dioxide is pushed out of the body.

Ok!...Let's begin breathing better.

INCORRECT BREATHING

Most people, when asked to sit up straight and breathe deeply, end up doing two things that are incorrect:

1 **Inhaling Incorrectly**
As they breathe in deeply, they expand the chest first, and they draw in the abdomen as they inhale.

2 **Exhaling Incorrectly**
As they exhale, they slouch forward with their chest and shoulders and their belly goes out.

Both of these are incorrect. This method of breathing in and out cheats all of the abdominal muscles and nerves and does not allow proper ventilation of the lungs.

"So I asked the neighbor lady next door, 'Take a deep breath for me and show me how you breathe deeply.' Well, she took a deep breath, and sure enough, she sucked in her stomach. And I said, 'You're breathing wrong.' She said, 'Well, how else would you breathe?' I showed her how you fill up your tummy first, then your chest, and so on. 'Oh,' she said, 'how do you do that?' So I showed her again. 'Then,' I said, 'you can even press it out with your hands if you can't do it with your muscles. And she said, 'Oh, my gosh!' At first she couldn't get it coordinated right, but she's getting the idea now, and she's beginning to learn. People usually suck in their stomachs when they breathe in deeply. I'm breathing so much better now, that it's hard for me to even do it that old way. It's wonderful!"

Jeanne Hrovat
66
Cleveland, Ohio

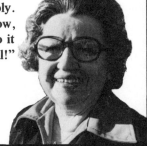

BREATHING EXERCISE 1 BELLY BREATH

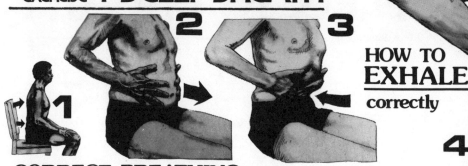

CORRECT BREATHING

HOW TO EXHALE. Sit up straight in your chair **(1)**. Do not lean against the back of the chair. Now put your hands on your belly as in illustration **(2)**. Spread your fingers wide apart so that you cover your belly area. Now press in firmly with your hands and fingers as in **(3)**, and as you press in, breathe out through your nose. **This means that you will be breathing out as you press your belly in (4).**

HOW TO INHALE. Now, as you breathe in, release your hands slowly, letting the belly drop down and out **(5)** as though it were being filled with air. **This means that you will be breathing in as your belly goes out.**

In order to see how this will look when it is done correctly, look right at the hands in Figure **(4)**. Now look at the hands in Figure **(5)**. Look back and forth quickly from **(4)** to **(5)** several times and you will see how the belly goes in and out.

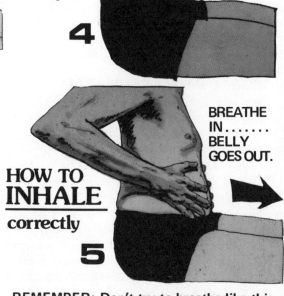

HOW TO EXHALE correctly

BREATHE OUT.....BELLY GOES IN..

HOW TO INHALE correctly

BREATHE IN.......BELLY GOES OUT.

REMEMBER: Don't try to breathe like this all day. Just do 2–5 minutes of breathing exercise every day, morning and evening.

BREATHING EXERCISE 2 BELLY BREATH against the wall

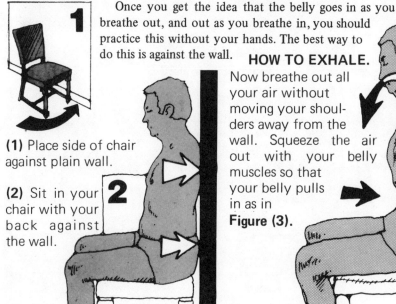

Once you get the idea that the belly goes in as you breathe out, and out as you breathe in, you should practice this without your hands. The best way to do this is against the wall.

(1) Place side of chair against plain wall.

(2) Sit in your chair with your back against the wall.

HOW TO EXHALE.
Now breathe out all your air without moving your shoulders away from the wall. Squeeze the air out with your belly muscles so that your belly pulls in as in **Figure (3)**.

HOW TO INHALE. Now breathe in and let your belly fill, relaxing outwards. Your belly should pull in as you exhale; relax down and out as you inhale. **Practice this 2-5 minutes morning and evening.**

83

BREATHING EXERCISE 3 COMPLETE BREATH

The quality of your breathing is completely dependent on how effectively your breathing muscles work. Doing Belly Breath forces you to use the belly muscles to squeeze the last bit of breath out. It also forces you to use the diaphragm muscle to inhale. Complete Breath goes one step further and brings the chest muscles, and even some shoulder muscles, into play. So, by doing Complete Breath, you are exercising all of your breathing muscles; this is like breath insurance helping you live a longer, healthier life.

HOW TO INHALE COMPLETELY In order to inhale, you slowly expand the belly and chest. This activates the diaphragm muscle and chest muscles, and pulls air into the lungs. To expand and lift the belly and chest completely requires slow, gentle effort.

HOW TO EXHALE COMPLETELY Exhalation, in Complete Breath, is primarily a relaxation process. After completely filling the lungs with air, the chest muscles in the rib cage and shoulders will be tense. In order to exhale, simply begin to slowly relax these muscles, and the air will begin to come out. You will notice a tendency to want to breathe out quickly as you exhale. You may

> **THE COMPLETE BREATH, EXERCISES ALL BREATHING MUSCLES.**
>
> Exercises all breathing muscles and nerves of the chest and rib cage.
>
> Exercises the diaphragm muscle and nerves.
>
> Exercises belly muscles and nerves.

also have a tendency to slump forward as you exhale. Both of these must be avoided. Instead, relax your chest slowly, controlling the exhalation so that it is slow and gradual. When you have relaxed your chest completely there will still be some air left inside, so continue to sit up straight and pull your belly in, squeezing the remainder of the air out of your lungs. **NOTE: Even though the air you breathe actually only enters the lungs, in Yoga you try to feel as though the air fills the entire body as you breathe. This makes the breathing process easier and more effective.**

Always breathe in and out through your nose.

Your nose warms and filters air before it gets to your lungs. When you exhale it is much easier for you to control your breath if you use your nose instead of your mouth.

HOW TO INHALE

To begin your Complete Breath exercise, sit up straight and exhale all air from your lungs so you can begin with a fresh inhalation.

3. Keep on inhaling until the air fills all the way to the top. It will feel as though the top of your chest is expanding and lifting as you finish filling the top of your lungs, **figure (3). Remember: As you fill the very top of your lungs, be careful not to draw your belly inward.**

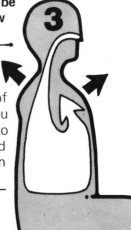

1. Now as you begin to inhale, relax your belly muscles slowly and feel as though you are filling your belly with air, as in **figure (1).**

2. After you have filled your belly, keep filling up into the middle of your chest. You will now begin to feel your chest and rib cage expand, as in **figure (2).**

84

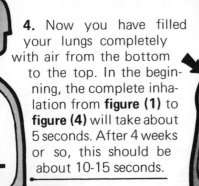

4. Now you have filled your lungs completely with air from the bottom to the top. In the beginning, the complete inhalation from **figure (1)** to **figure (4)** will take about 5 seconds. After 4 weeks or so, this should be about 10-15 seconds.

FULL UP

HOW TO EXHALE

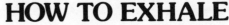

5. After you have inhaled completely, as in **figure (4)**, hold your breath in for just a brief moment, and then begin immediately to exhale as slowly as possible. In order to exhale, all you have to do is begin to let the air out slowly, as in **figure (5). Don't let the air come rushing out; instead, control it, exhaling gently and slowly.**

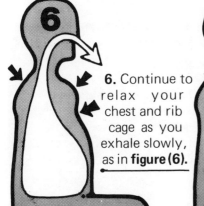

6. Continue to relax your chest and rib cage as you exhale slowly, as in **figure (6).**

7. After you have relaxed your chest and rib cage, there is still a lot of air left in your lungs, so begin to pull your belly in just like you do in Belly Breath, **figure (7).** This will force the remaining breath out. **Remember: Do not slouch forward as you pull the belly in.**

•Daily Practice•

After you have finished breathing in completely and breathing out completely, just continue this quiet process of completely filling and emptying the lungs. Close your eyes and concentrate on your breathing to the exclusion of everything else. Feel everything you can about breathing. Relax your face and your mind, and just observe the breath flowing in and out of your body. Feel this subtle energy of breath that everything in life depends upon. Continue practicing this breathing exercise for 2-5 minutes in the morning and evening. Within a month you will be able to do this for 5-10 minutes. You'll love it and feel calm and refreshed afterwards!

BREATHING EXERCISE 4 HUMMING BREATH

This is one of the very best exercises to strengthen the Humming Breath system. Again, you can't slouch forward as you breathe out. Sit up straight and use your muscles. In *Humming Breath* you fill your belly and chest in the same way as you do in Complete Breath, however, you sing the sound *hum* out as you exhale.

HOW TO INHALE ▪▪▪▪▪▪ HOW TO EXHALE ▪▪▪▪▪

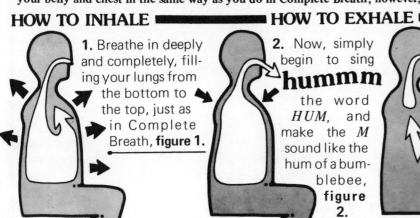

1. Breathe in deeply and completely, filling your lungs from the bottom to the top, just as in Complete Breath, **figure 1.**

2. Now, simply begin to sing **hummm** the word *HUM*, and make the *M* sound like the hum of a bumblebee, **figure 2.**

3. Sit up straight. Keep making that *humming* sound as long as possible. Pull your stomach **hummmmmmm** muscles in, squeezing out a few more seconds of that *humming* sound. Then relax the belly, breathe in fully, and do it again. Practice this for 2—3 minutes.

BREATHING EXERCISE 5 RELAXING BREATH

The Relaxing Breath is most beneficial in relaxing tensions at the end of the day and helping you get to sleep. Many people who experience insomnia say that this breathing exercise has helped them get to sleep without drugs.

Lie on your back comfortably. Spread your feet and lean your knees against each other. Place your hands on your belly and breathe in and out deeply and slowly, as in Complete Breath. **Your belly should rise as you inhale and drop down as you exhale.** Focus your attention on the sound and feeling of breathing to the exclusion of everything else. Relax all body and mind tensions more and more each time you exhale.

RELAX AS YOU EXHALE

BREATHING EXERCISE 6 STOMACH LIFT

The Stomach Lift breathing exercise is one of the most beneficial exercises an older person can do. This exercise alone could help older people to avoid numerous illnesses and diseases of their vital organs as well as completely eliminating debilitating constipation.

This exercise develops great control and strength in the nerves and muscles of the abdomen. Begin with one or two attempts per day, building up to 3–5 repetitions. When you reach 3–5 repetitions, try to hold the Number 3 position for a little longer, but do not exceed 5–7 seconds. This can be done on the floor or on your bed.

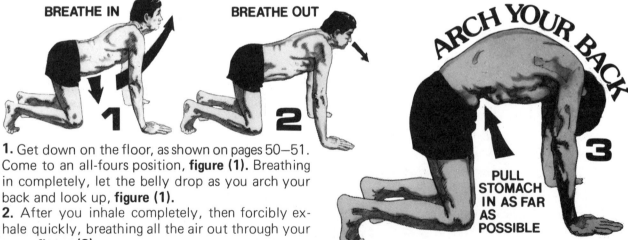

BREATHE IN

BREATHE OUT

ARCH YOUR BACK

PULL STOMACH IN AS FAR AS POSSIBLE

1. Get down on the floor, as shown on pages 50–51. Come to an all-fours position, **figure (1).** Breathing in completely, let the belly drop as you arch your back and look up, **figure (1).**

2. After you inhale completely, then forcibly exhale quickly, breathing all the air out through your nose, **figure (2).**

3. Then after you've exhaled completely and quickly, hold your breath out. Do not breathe in immediately. Instead, push down on the floor with your arms and shoulders and arch your back. As you do this, pull the belly up and in as far as possible and hold this position, **figure (3),** from 2–5 seconds.

4. Then relax your belly and let it drop down. As you do this, relax down out of the arched position. After returning to **position (1),** breathe in deeply and relax. **Begin with 2 or 3 repetitions. Build up to 3–5 repetitions over a month's daily practice.**

RELAXATION & MEDITATION SECTION 8

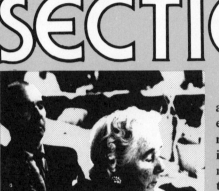

Taking a few minutes every day to relax and meditate gives you a refreshing vacation from the exhausting mental replay of petty emotional upsets. Americans traditionally take so little time for reflection and silence that this aspect of EDY training is often intensely meaningful. Relaxation and meditation help us learn more about ourselves by giving us an effective technique to control the wanderings of the mind. This allows you to become aware of beautiful parts of yourself that you may not have been aware of before, as well as helping to reduce physical stress and anxiety.

THE NEED FOR RELAXATION

Americans spend $72.6 billion every year on recreation. Much of our frantic rush to enjoy ourselves is based on a physical and mental need for relaxation and a fear of being quiet and alone with ourselves. Tension has become the curse of modern society,

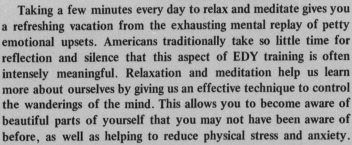

and few of us know how to deal with it effectively. In fact, the conspicuous consumption of alcohol and tranquilizers among the elderly indicates that this group of Americans may have the biggest need for positive ways to relieve tension.

The EDY relaxation technique is a step-by-step mental inventory of the body. While lying on the bed or the floor, or sitting in a comfortable position, students learn to mentally visualize and relax each part of the body. The process takes about five minutes and can be learned by anyone. These five minutes of conscious resting are as refreshing as a half-hour nap.

The results of this deceptively simple technique are truly remarkable. Relaxation procedures have been applied thera-

Americans spend $72.6 Billion dollars on recreation every year.

peutically in hospitals and outpatient treatment centers to alleviate chronic body and back pain, hypertension, anxiety, and other disorders. Many of us suffer from these common problems. You can safely apply the EDY self-help relaxation program to your specific needs in your own home. Students report that they practice the technique to elimi-

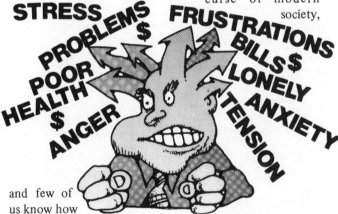

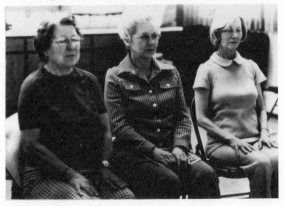

nate insomnia, and many tell us that through daily practice they have reduced their dependence on alcohol, tranquilizers, and sedatives. The conscious removal of muscle tension every day also helps to eliminate tension headaches and reduce annoying body aches and pains. Students also report that they are less anxious and irritable and that they therefore get along better with their friends and family. In addition, they report renewed sexual vigor. Since anxiety and stress are major causes of hypertension (high blood pressure), many of our students have also found that their daily relaxation routine has significantly reduced their blood pressure worries.

MEDITATION
A QUIET REFLECTIVE MOMENT IN YOUR DAY.

Meditation is a calm silencing of the mind which develops concentration and increased mental clarity. The first step is thorough relaxation of the body and breathing. After the relaxation procedure, students concentrate on keeping their mind still and motionless for 10–15 minutes.

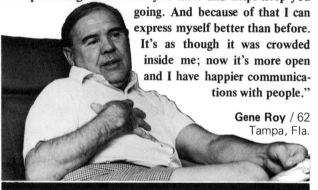

"It clears up your thinking, your mind. You just shut your eyes and relax, and it stops everything from moving so fast, it really does. You just feel that there's more joy in you, it's so peaceful, and that relaxed feeling that you had while you were practicing comes over you later and helps keep you going. And because of that I can express myself better than before. It's as though it was crowded inside me; now it's more open and I have happier communications with people."

Gene Roy / 62
Tampa, Fla.

The meditative state of restful alertness is unlike sleeping or daydreaming. You remain conscious and aware throughout, gently letting go of all mental activity. This helps you to become totally quiet and self-observant.

EDY meditation is a practical mental discipline which brings about increased will power and greater sensitivity to the beauty of living. It helps you to enjoy your life more. As an older person, now is the best time for you to make a concerted attempt to find what is real and lasting about the world and yourself. The cool, detached observation of the meditative mind is the best perspective from which to see these things.

The practice of EDY meditation, by creating a quiet, reflective moment in your day, increases your self-understanding. You learn how to amplify what you like about yourself and how to discard those parts of your personality that your are not so happy with—such as unnecessary anger and childish behavior patterns. As you become more aware of your inner self and the depth and beauty inside, you will tend to feel better about yourself. This will enable you to be happy when you are by yourself and reduce your feelings of boredom, fear, and loneliness. EDY meditation also improves your intuition, making your hunches more reliable. Most importantly, EDY meditation practice yields the wisdom to know your true desires and purpose in life. This knowledge allows you to stand proudly and guide the following generations.

YOGA IS NOT A RELIGION.

Meditation, the basic component of classical Yoga, is at least 5,000 years old. Although the meditation techniques of classical Yoga were adopted into Hinduism, Buddhism, Jainism, and many other world religions, classical Yoga is much older and is a distinct philosophic and psychological approach to self-awareness. Meditation is a technique which clarifies your perception of yourself and the world through the development of an intuitive, uncluttered mind. If you wish, you can use your Yoga meditation to enhance and intensify your chosen faith.

OK!...Let's begin to meditate.

In your Easy Does It Yoga training you will learn a Complete Relaxation procedure as well as two meditation techniques.

The Complete Relaxation is a quiet process of visualizing your entire body and systematically relaxing any and all tensions in your muscles, nerves, and vital organs. This process is extremely enjoyable, and after you learn and practice it for a while, you'll be able to relax and relieve tensions throughout the day. After you release all body tensions through your Complete Relaxation procedure, your body will seem to relax and disappear slightly, almost

as though you forget about it for a while. It is at this point that Yoga meditation begins. You will have a choice of two different meditation techniques to employ after your Complete Relaxation procedure. Yoga meditation is not a process of self-analyzation; in fact, the less you talk to yourself during meditation, the better your experience will be.

The main objective of Yoga meditation is to get a clear, more comprehensive understanding of yourself. All of the curative physiological effects, such as reduced high blood pressure, alpha brain waves, reduced lactic acid in the blood, etc., are all actually side effects of the main objective.

6 helpful hints for better meditation

There are a few very basic rules to abide by during your meditation training.
If you follow these closely, you will learn this subtle process faster and easier.

1 Do not do your meditation after a heavy meal, as this will inhibit blood flow to the brain and reduce your ability to quiet the mind.

2 Don't meditate with your pets. They may jump on your lap or otherwise disturb you while you are in a very quiet state, and this may startle you.

3 For the same reason, take the phone off the hook and let your family and friends know not to disturb you for just a few minutes while you do your meditation.

4 Do not try too hard—too much strain and effort will keep you from relaxing. Don't worry if you fall asleep; this is normal. After continued practice you will not fall asleep and will be able to remain alert.

5 Don't try to meditate and relax after drinking a lot of coffee or tea, or while under the influence of alcohol. These will make your heart rate change and this will impede your total relaxation of body and mind.

6 Try to practice at the same time every day.

YOUR COMPLETE RELAXATION PROCEDURE
A gradual & systematic way to release tensions & get complete rest.

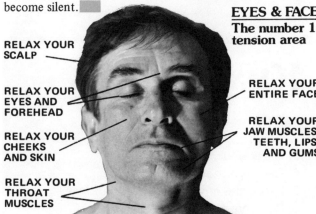

PALMS UP

LET FEET RELAX

EYES & FACE
The number 1 tension area

RELAX YOUR SCALP

RELAX YOUR EYES AND FOREHEAD

RELAX YOUR CHEEKS AND SKIN

RELAX YOUR THROAT MUSCLES

RELAX YOUR ENTIRE FACE

RELAX YOUR JAW MUSCLES, TEETH, LIPS, AND GUMS

RELAX YOUR ARMS UNTIL THEY FEEL EMPTY

Lie down flat on your back with your arms alongside your body, palms up. Let your legs relax so that your feet fall apart slightly. **OPTIONS:** You may place a small pillow under your head or under the back of your knees to relieve any discomfort in the lower back. You may also do this on your bed or on your mat on the floor. Do not get chilled—throw a blanket or a shawl over you to stay warm. Now, mentally remind yourself that for 10–15 minutes you are going to completely relax and become silent.

Focus your attention quietly on each part of the body and visualize it as we go along. Start with your face. Gently and calmly bring all of your attention to your forehead. Feel all of the muscles in your forehead. Now let them relax so they become loose. Now be aware of how your eyes feel. Are they tense and jittery? The eyes are usually the hardest part of the body to relax, so just let them loosen and float in the eye sockets. You aren't going to use your eyes now, so let all tenseness and movement in the eyes stop. Don't tense them, relax and quiet them. Move on to your lips, teeth, and all the muscles of the jaw, mouth, and throat. Let your tongue relax in your mouth, and say to yourself, "I don't have to speak now for a few minutes." Let all the skin on your face become very loose and still. Let your scalp relax and let your ears droop towards the floor. Your eyes may continue to jump around a little, but don't worry—after some regular practice you will be able to relax them more and more.

Now let's relax the shoulders, arms, and hands. Feel as though you are inside of your arms and that they are hollow inside. Let all the muscles of the shoulders settle loosely on the floor. Now move down into your elbow joints and imagine you can see and feel the bones. Let them relax and loosen. Now move down into your forearms, wrists, and right into your hands and fingers, making them hollow, loose, and empty. Relax your fingers completely as though they are empty gloves lying on a table. Now silently move your attention, like a tiny, warm relaxing beam of light, into your chest, and for a few moments, just observe the air moving in and out of your lungs. Feel your heart beating softly and rhythmically, and notice your belly rising and falling as you breathe. Do not make any attempt to speed up or slow down your breathing. Instead, picture your lungs—take in a nice gentle breath of air, and just as though you are sighing, let the breath out and relax your lungs. Take in another deep, gentle breath, sigh it out, and feel as though your heart also relaxes. Then just let go of your breathing altogether, and relax all tension or effort in your breathing. Observe your belly and try to relax the squeezing effort as you breathe out. Each time you exhale,

YOUR COMPLETE RELAXATION PROCEDURE
A gradual & systematic way to release tensions & get complete rest.

BREATHING The number 2 tension area

RELAX YOUR BREATHING AND
YOUR HEART

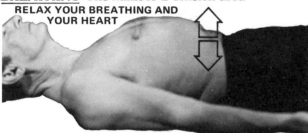

relax the squeezing of your breath a little more, making it as relaxed as possible so that you are exerting almost no effort or strain to breathe.

RELAX YOUR THIGHS, KNEES, AND FEET, MAKING THEM FEEL EMPTY

Next, move your attention down into your legs, and make your legs hollow and empty, just as you did with the arms. Loosen and relax your thighs, hip sockets, and groin. Let your legs completely relax and cease moving. Imagine that you are inside of your thighs and they are hollow. Relax your knee joints and feel as though the lower leg is also hollow and empty, all the way into your toes. Imagine your feet are empty with nothing inside, not even any bones. Feel as though your toenails relax and loosen.

Now move up your empty feet, legs, and thighs silently, and bring your attention to the base of your spine. Feel your spine and all of its joints from the base of your spine up to the base of your skull at the back of your neck. As you move upwards through your waist area, relax any sign of tension so that your entire spine loosens. When you get to the top of your spine in your neck, spend a little extra time at this spot. It is a tension site and needs a little extra relaxation. So relax all muscles and

NECK & SHOULDERS The number 3 tension area

tension at the back of your neck where your spine connects to your head. Imagine you can look right down inside of your spinal column as though your spine were a rope dangling down into a dark well. Relax your spine so much that it feels loose like that rope dangling down into the well.

RELAX THE BACK OF YOUR NECK AND RECHECK YOUR FACE AND EYES FOR TENSION

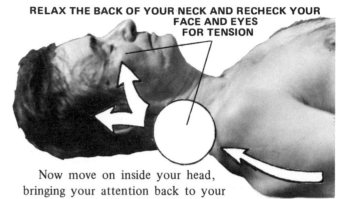

Now move on inside your head, bringing your attention back to your face to see whether or not your face is tense. Let go of your eyes even more now, and let them float almost as though you can't feel them move at all. You can relax your eyes the same way you can when you tense and relax your hands completely.

Now before we go on to the next stage, you should quietly observe the whole inside of your body from head to toe. Recheck the three main tension areas. 1) Is your breathing relaxed? 2) Are your eyes and facial muscles relaxed? 3) Is the back of your neck relaxed? Your body will eventually feel as though it is just an empty shell with no tension anywhere. The only movement left will be your heart and your breathing, but they also will be very relaxed. Now relax the entire inside of your head. Feel as though it quietly settles inside your head with no effort or strain—just quiet and still.

This is the demarcation point between your Complete Relaxation procedure and the beginning of your meditation technique.

10 STEPS TO COMPLETE RELAXATION

1. Relax your face and eyes.
2. Relax and empty your arms and hands.
3. Relax your lungs and heart.
4. Relax your belly and breathing.
5. Relax and empty your legs and feet.
6. Relax your lower back and spine.
7. Relax and loosen your upper back, shoulders, and neck.
8. Relax the inside of your head.
9. Recheck the three major tension areas: 1) your face and eyes; 2) your breathing; 3) the back of your neck.
10. Quietly begin your mental meditation.

OM MEDITATION TECHNIQUE

THE MEDITATIVE ABILITY TO FOCUS AND RELAX THE MIND WITH THE SOUND OM.

Your first meditation procedure, OM Meditation, uses a specific meditation sound that you repeat over and over again to yourself mentally. Meditation sounds are called "mantrums." There are hundreds of meditational sounds that Yogis have used for thousands of years to center and focus the wandering and scattered mind and its energies. The mantrum we recommend for your use is the oldest and most basic mantrum in classical Yoga—OM. The OM mantrum of classical Yoga was adopted and used in a religious way by nearly every religion of the Eastern world to signify one thing or another in their particular faith and theology. However, in classical Yoga, the mantrum OM is used as a purely psychological tool, like a musical note, to center and focus the mind and is not meant to indicate any particular religious concept or deity.

Yogis say that if you could hear the subtle humming sound of the collective atomic structure of your own body and mind, that sound would most resemble the sound OM.

The purely psychological aspects of Om were delineated more than 2,500 years ago in the *Manduka Upanishad* where the sound Om is interpreted allegorically to possess four distinct elements pertaining to four different states of consciousness. The first part of the sound OM signifies our **conscious self** when we are awake. The second part signifies our **subconscious self,** when we are asleep and dreaming. The third aspect of OM, the *M* sound, has to do with our **unconscious self,** when we are in deep dreamless sleep; and the fourth aspect of the sound OM signifies that portion of ourselves that exists in absolute silence of mind in what is called our **"witness consciousness."** Hence, by the repetition and focusing upon the sound OM, one's mind is led gently into a timeless peace and silence beyond description. This, in classical Yoga, is a purely psychological process designed to give us knowledge of our own self.

How is this done ?

After you have gone through your body relaxing and releasing any tensions or constrictions, then your body will become intensely still and calm. After you have brought your attention back up to your head and double checked your facial/eye tension, then gently begin to repeat the sound OM over and over again to yourself; not out loud, but mentally. The sound OM sounds like the word HOME if you leave off the H and the E. Simply relax deeper and deeper, repeating this sound over and over to yourself mentally for 10–15 minutes.

At first... you will be repeating the sound OM mentally, and the next moment your mental voice will start talking about some completely unrelated idea or thought. In fact, your mind may babble on for quite a long time before you realize that you're not repeating OM any longer. For example, it may sound like this:

OM OM OM OM **Oh my goodness, I forgot to pay the phone bill. That reminds me, I'd better call. . . .**

After some practice... you will notice that your mind wanders away from OM and starts talking about something else. Bring it back to OM gently and start repeating OM again. Your mind will jump off to other ideas

quite frequently in the beginning as it is not used to focusing on one thing for any length of time; therefore, it wanders about from one thing to the next. Don't be discouraged by this. It happens to everyone. Also don't worry if, in the beginning, you forget completely about what you were doing and fall asleep. Do not fight your mind or chastise yourself when you discover that instead of meditation on the sound OM you're planning out what to feed your cat or some other completely unrelated idea. Instead, gently return to OM as soon as you realize that you're talking about something else. It may help you to imagine that you're listening to OM on the radio and suddenly the channel switches to a soap opera, or news, etc. Instead of yelling about it, simply return the mental channel to the sound OM and continue as though nothing happened. For example, it may sound like this:

OM OM OM OM OM OM **What should I wear to lunch today** OM OM OM **I hope the car starts easier today than it did yesterday** OM OM OM **Boy, that argument with Sarah yesterday really upset me. Hope she's not mad at me!** OM OM. . . . .

Your ability to focus gently and effortlessly on the repetition of the sound OM will improve so that fewer ideas and thoughts disrupt your relaxed concentration, and instead of the long mental dialogues that used to go on and on in your mind, now they're shorter, and it may sound like this:

OM OM OM OM OM OM OM OM OM OM OM OM OM OM **Wonder what time it is** OM OM OM OM OM OM OM OM OM OM OM OM **Hope my check comes today** OM OM OM OM OM OM OM OM OM

After regular daily practice...

In fact, your ability to focus on the sound OM will become almost effortless, and you will be able to continue the sound mentally with virtually no disruptions for minutes on end, whereas before you might hardly have been able to repeat three or five OM's without the mind wandering. Sometimes even the OM sound will relax into silence for a while, and then start up again. This will feel wonderful to you and it will sound like this:

OM OM OM OM OM OM OM OM OM OM OM OM OM OM OM OM OM ...silence...OM OM OM OM

Coming out of meditation...

Coming out of meditation is as important as how you relax into it. If you get up too quickly, or disturb yourself too abruptly, it may make you jittery or upset. So to insure against this happening, take a couple of minutes to awaken your body and mind to activity again. Don't just jump up. Increase your breathing first, and that will start to reactivate everything else. At first, when you go to move your hands and arms, they may feel a little like wood since they've become so utterly relaxed. Stretch your arms and legs like a cat does when it awakens from a rest period. Then just lie there for a moment and get used to moving again. After a couple minutes you can get up and move into your active life again, refreshed, alert, and recharged with new energy and a clear mind.

> Each Meditation Practice Period should consist of 5–10 minutes of your Complete Relaxation plus 10–15 minutes of either your OM Meditation or SAT Meditation technique. You have just learned your OM Meditation, now continue and learn the SAT Meditation technique.

SAT-SILENT AWARENESS TRAINING
THE ABILITY TO EXTEND MEDITATIVE AWARENESS INTO PURE MENTAL SILENCE.

Although both meditation techniques are done right after your Complete Relaxation procedure, SAT Meditation (pronounced so it rhymes with "hot") differs from OM Meditation in a distinct way. Instead of focusing your mind on the sound OM, in SAT Meditation you begin to listen to your Mental Dialogue babbling on and on in your mind.

As you do this you will become aware of occasional silent gaps, or moments between thoughts and mental dialogue. These are moments of pure mental silence when one idea has finished and another has yet to begin. Focusing on these silent moments between thoughts is for some people easier than focusing upon a continuously repeated sound, while some people find OM Meditation easier than SAT. You should try both and choose the one you like best.

Both SAT and OM Meditation techniques are similar in that in either technique the mind will at first jump about. In OM Meditation the mind will wander away from OM to other thoughts and ideas. In SAT Meditation the mind will babble on and on in a seemingly endless dialogue. A silent moment will finally appear, and as you attempt to retain it silently, all of a sudden the mental talking will start up again and off you go into another idea. It may make it a bit clearer if you realize that in OM Meditation you are trying to hear the continuous gentle repetition of the sound OM to the exclusion of everything else, whereas in SAT Meditation you are attempting to hear silence of the mind for longer and longer periods of time to the exclusion of any mental dialogue whatsoever.

How is this done ?
At first... After finishing your Complete Relaxation procedure and rechecking the three major tension areas, then just forget all about your body and quietly begin to listen for your own mental voice talking to yourself. Soon you will begin to hear your mental voice talking. You can listen to your mind talk and it goes on and on in a seemingly endless babble. It may sound something like this:

Well now....I'm going to be quiet now....Gee, I hope the phone doesn't ring....That reminds me, I've got to call Mary about lunch....Oh, what will I wear...maybe that new hat?...No, maybe...

After some practice... Trying to force your mind to be quiet will only increase the mental talking. However, **you can separate yourself from its seemingly**

endless prattle by shifting your attention. As you are lying there quietly listening to your mind, begin to listen and wait for your mental voice to finish the idea and sentence that it is engaged in. Wait calmly and patiently, and soon your mental voice will complete the sentence, and at that very moment, you will notice a pause, a silent moment before the mental voice begins talking again. It may sound like this:

Don't forget to get the car fixed. Gotta call the garage and make an appointment . . .SILENCE . . .

In SAT Meditation you must first become aware of the fact that although the mind seems to ramble on and on endlessly, in reality there are gaps of silence as one idea ends and the next has yet to begin. And since there are many ideas coming and going all the time in your mind, so are there numerous silent moments between thoughts and mental talk. Listen carefully, and as the mental voice finishes talking for a moment, try to retain that silent moment a little longer. **While you are in that silent moment you should not hear your mental voice say anything at all.** Try to stay in that silence, and for a moment or two you will be absolutely still and quiet with no sound, no thought, and no movement of the mind, yet you will remain alert, aware, and blissfully silent. It's kind of like slipping across the street between the rush of heavy traffic. You move into silence in the space between one thought and the next.

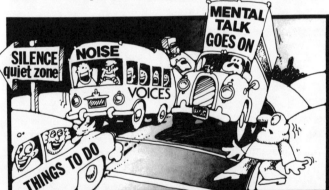

In the beginning this moment of silence will only last a moment before the mind starts talking again. Don't be upset by this. Wait and listen, and you'll soon notice that this new idea soon ends and another gap of silence appears. Again and again your mental voice will break the silence, and again and again you wait for the next silent moment. It may sound like this:

Gee, the kids haven't called in so long. . . . . . .I hope everything's all right with them. Oh, they must be, or they'd surely call. . . .SILENCE . . . Can't forget Dorothy's birthday. If I send her present this week it'll surely get there in time for her party on the 5th. . . . . .SILENCE . . . .

After regular daily practice...

After just a few days' practice you'll begin to gain the ability to let go of mental dialogue effortlessly and rest blissfully between thought and mental dialogue in a timeless silence of mind. In the beginning the silent moments between mental conversations only lasted a brief moment; however, with some daily practice, you will find that you can slip into and hold these silent moments for longer periods of time, like this:

Gee, I wonder what I'd feel like if I didn't say anything at all to myself? . . . . . .SILENCE . . . . .CONTINUED SILENCE. . . . . .Boy, is it quiet. . . . . .SILENCE. wonder what time it is. . . . . . . .SILENCE . . . .

Again and again the mental voice will start talking, and again and again you wait for the idea to finish and then let go again into silence. With regular practice you will even be able to let go into silence right in the middle of a word or sentence that the mental voice is taking about, like this . . .

Gee, if only I could stop talki . . . . SILENCE. . . . .

Coming out of meditation

Be sure not to move too rapidly coming out of meditation. Move slowly and gently and take a few minutes to reactivate—the same way you did at the end of your OM Meditation procedure.

"My husband died four years ago, and I've been alone since. Last week I had an appointment with a lawyer to make out a will of my own. I was worried that it might be upsetting, so I did my meditation before I got cleaned up to go. And you know, it seemed as though my meditation relaxed me enough that the lawyer thing didn't upset me. Any other time I'm sure that type of thing would have bothered me, but it didn't. I really was surprised."

Pauline Moody
73
Bradenton,
Florida

SEATED MEDITATION

YOUR SEATED RELAXATION PROCEDURE

After first learning to relax and meditate lying down, you will then want to learn to relax and meditate seated in a chair.

Before beginning either OM Meditation or SAT in the seated position, you should go through your body and gradually relax any tensions or constrictions, the same as you do lying down.

How is this done?

Sit up erect and comfortably in your chair. You may support your back against the chair back, but **do not slouch.** Seated meditation is particularly effective right after your seated breathing exercises. Now you follow the same Complete Relaxation procedure as you learned lying down. Begin at your face, move down to the feet, and then return up the spine into the head. The main objective of your Seated Relaxation procedure is not only to relax the body completely, but also to sit as motionless as possible. Relaxed motionlessness of your body will make your meditation very easy and pleasant. It will help if during your relaxation procedure you spend a little extra time relaxing the three major tension areas.

THE ABILITY TO SIT MOTIONLESS

Complete Relaxation procedures and meditation produce what we call a Minimal Tension State, wherein the body is almost completely motionless except, of course, for breathing and heart action, and the mind also becomes motionless and silent. The ability to achieve this state of being will put you in harmony with nature's own cycles of activity followed by rest. To achieve total fitness one must learn how to be active as well as how to be still; thus your entire being benefits. By decreasing physical movements during meditation training, the body and its nerves rest in a way better than sleep. This also frees the mind from the body, allowing it to recharge and develop new abilities of thinking and perceiving.

1. Relax your face & eyes.

You always begin with relaxing your facial muscles, your eyes and forehead. You then move on into the rest of the body and then recheck your face and eyes again at the end of your relaxation procedure before beginning your meditation procedure. The important thing is to relax your eyes and forehead so much that you no longer feel them move or constrict.

2. Relax your breathing.

Then don't forget to focus your attention upon the squeezing out of the breath as you exhale. Try to relax this squeezing tension until your breath becomes easy and effortless.

3. Relax the back of your neck.

Relax the back of your neck. And as you move back up your back, focus your attention in the neck region and ease any remaining tension so that your head feels loose and balanced on top of your neck and shoulders. Be especially alert to tensions right up under the base of the skull where the neck joins the head.

Now you're ready to begin either OM Meditation or SAT. Meditate for 10–15 minutes and don't forget to move slowly as you come out of meditation.

Ok...now what?

OK! Now you're ready to begin meditating on a regular daily basis. For the first week, practice your Complete Relaxation procedure (5–10 minutes), followed by your OM Meditation (10–15 minutes). In the second week do your Complete Relaxation (5–10 minutes), followed by your Silent Awareness Training (10–15 minutes). Then after trying each one for one week, choose the one you like the best and practice it alone for three months. After becoming proficient and comfortable with either OM or SAT Meditation, you can then begin to try the other technique occasionally. After first learning to meditate lying down you can then learn it sitting up. In one year you will have a wide range of meditation procedures that will fit any and all needs and circumstances.

● **You might even take your book and read some of the Relaxation and Meditation instructions into a tape recorder and play it back to help you practice. If you don't want to do this yourself, you can purchase these Relaxation and Meditation instructions from us in cassette tapes. Write The Light of Yoga Society at the address on page 112 for cassette tape prices and listings.**

DAILY ROUTINES SECTION 9

This is the most important section in the book for those of you who are wanting to begin a daily practice of Easy Does It Yoga. It is in this section that you'll find an easy beginning routine of daily exercise, breathing, and meditation, as well as a schedule for better nutrition and philosophical study. Although this routine only covers your first six weeks of practice, by the time you finish it you will have a thorough understanding of the basic principles and procedures of EDY. You will then be able to incorporate a variety of the one hundred different techniques in this book into your own personal routine.

CAUTIONS & HINTS

Please read and follow these cautions and hints carefully and you will progress rapidly and safely in your practice of Easy Does It Yoga.

CAUTIONS

1. In any program of exercise—no matter how well designed—there is a possibility of injury, especially if you haven't exercised in a long time. This fact should not inhibit you from trying; we just ask that you use your good common sense. Begin gently and avoid strain and over-zealousness.

2. If you have a history of heart trouble, spinal injury, high blood pressure, chronic arthritis, or some other serious ailment or injury; or if you are on heavy medication, please take this book to your doctor to help you design a routine that will be compatible with your limitations.

3. Do not do these exercises while under the influence of alcohol.

4. Wait 1½–2 hours after a heavy meal before exercising or meditating.

5. Don't try to do your breathing and meditation right after drinking a lot of tea or coffee.

HINTS

1. Try to practice at the same time every day if possible. Choose a time when you will be the least disturbed by your family, friends, pets, or telephone.

2. Do not tense your facial muscles during exercise or breathing techniques. Keep your face relaxed.

3. Read the breathing instructions carefully for each exercise and follow them exactly.

4. Don't strain by doing more repetitions than are recommended. Read the instructions carefully and follow the procedures exactly.

5. Use a chair for support and balance. This will really help you improve quickly.

6. Don't strain too hard at any of this—Easy Does It!

7. Don't exercise or meditate in a cold draft.

8. Exercising after a warm bath or shower can help you loosen up, but be sure to stay warm.

9. Always breathe through your nose while doing the breathing techniques and exercises.

10. Always approach your exercises with a calm, gentle approach and avoid any bouncing or jerky movements that may be injurious.

THE BEST TIME OF DAY

The best time of day to do your Yoga routine is **whenever it is most convenient** for you. Some people like to do their exercises first thing in the morning, while others prefer late morning before lunch. Many people like the late afternoon or evening, while others prefer to do theirs just before going to bed. It doesn't matter when you do them, as long as you do them regularly—even for just a few minutes a day, every day.

YOUR BIGGEST PROBLEM?

The biggest problem that most people experience is being regular in their daily practice. **Set aside the same time of day for your Yoga and try to stick with it every day**. It is better to do 10 or 15 minutes of practice every day, than miss 4 or 5 days, and then try to catch up. If you do miss a few days, don't get discouraged, just try again.

UNDER THE WEATHER ROUTINE

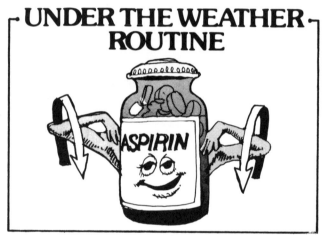

Now, because of Easy Does It Yoga, even if you have to rest in bed due to illness, you can still do a few simple exercises that will help you remain active and recuperate faster. For instance, if you have a cold or the flu, you may not be able to do your breathing and standing exercises, but you can still do the **shoulder/arm exercises on pages 33—38**. You might even be able to do several of the **bed exercises on pages 67—70**. Many of these exercises will also help you to relieve bed sores and constipation. You can almost always do your **meditation and relaxation** procedures in **Section 8**.

Don't forget, if your're ill, you need to take extra care of your **nutrition**. Vitamins and minerals, especially Vitamin C, will help you to recuperate faster. **See pages 106—107**. Also, you might use this time more constructively by catching up on your **philosophical study. See pages 108—111**.

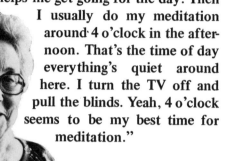

"I practice 15—20 minutes of EDY exercise first thing in the morning before breakfast, and that helps me get going for the day. Then I usually do my meditation around 4 o'clock in the afternoon. That's the time of day everything's quiet around here. I turn the TV off and pull the blinds. Yeah, 4 o'clock seems to be my best time for meditation."

Alice Blauvelt
66
Bradenton, Florida

A POSITIVE ATTITUDE

A positive, supportive, creative attitude about your practices and life are a major addition and uplifting factor in EDY. A doctor once told Swami Rama, "You aren't getting any younger, you know. You shouldn't walk so fast—slow down." Rama's reply was, "Young man, when I'm dead and let go of this body, maybe then it will slow down; until then I will remain active!" A positive attitude will help to support you and boost your moods and self-assurance. Besides, it feels better to be positive than negative, depressed, and hopeless. Rama also said, "Even in the face of the most dreadful calamities, a positive attitude is better than a negative one." Also, it's infectious, and one person being bright and positive helps others too.

UP& AT IT!

Well, this is it. **It's time to get up and get at it!** So get a towel, blanket, or exercise mat for you to exercise on. **Keep this blanket or mat reserved just for your Yoga.** Wear loose warm clothing that will not constrict or inhibit your movements. Remember: Yoga is not calisthenics. When you do the exercises, breathe as instructed, move slowly, hold the positions steady, and don't bounce or jerk. Now you're ready to begin, so turn the page. **Read your routines and enjoy!**

THE TOTAL YOU
YOUR DAILY ROUTINE FOR TOTAL FITNESS

In order to get the most effect from your Easy Does It Yoga, your daily practice should include some exercise, breathing, meditation, nutritional improvements, and philosophical study. This will enhance the total health of your body, mind, emotions, and spirit. The best daily routine should ideally consist of the following five areas of practice:

1 YOUR MAIN ROUTINE

You should have a **Main Routine** of EDY Exercise, Breathing, and Meditation that takes about 20—45 minutes. You should do this **Main Routine** once every day—*morning or evening.*

A suggested Main Routine:
YOGA EXERCISE —— **10—20 minutes**
Followed by . . .
YOGA BREATHING —— **5—10 minutes**
Followed by . . .
YOGA MEDITATION —**10—20 minutes**

2 YOUR MINI ROUTINE

Your **Main Routine** of 20—45 minutes of EDY can be done any time of day. Separate from your **Main Routine** you should also do a **Mini Routine:**

YOGA BREATHING ———— **5 minutes**
Followed by . . .
YOGA MEDITATION —**10—20 minutes**

SUGGESTION: If you do your **Main Routine** in the late morning before lunch, do your **Mini Routine** in the late afternoon or evening before dinner.

3 ANYTIME EXERCISES

In addition to your Main and Mini Routines you should also be trying to do some of the bed exercises first thing in the morning to get started and maybe some Relaxing Breath and Meditation last thing at night. Don't forget to do some exercises in your chair while watching TV and some deep breathing while you take a walk or ride your bike, or even your Silent Awareness Training while you wait in the dentist's office. **Do what you can, where you can. Be creative!**

4 NUTRITION TRAINING

In addition to your daily routines of EDY Exercise, Breathing, and Meditation, you should also see if you can come up with creative ways to improve your own nutrition, diet, and health by becoming more aware of the value of the foods you eat.

Read, study, and apply the information in **Section 10, Nutrition,** especially:
- **What You Can Do To Help Yourself**
- **7 Ways To Eat Less Bad Food & More Good Food**
- **Menus & Eating Tips**

5 YOUR STUDY ROUTINE

To round out your daily routine you should begin to study again. Try to consciously widen the viewpoints and concepts that you live by. Study subjects that you're not already familiar with.

Read, study, and apply Section 11, Philosophy:
- Try the **5 Ways to Increase Personal Growth.**
- **Form a study group and begin to read, study, and discuss the books and subjects in the suggested reading list on page 111.**

THE TOTAL YOU
YOUR DAILY ROUTINE FOR TOTAL FITNESS

This is your daily routine for the total fitness of the total you. It covers all five areas of Easy Does It Yoga and will give you a safe, gentle beginning that will make you feel wonderful. **Remember:** Read each week's routine through completely before beginning. Note that each exercise has a page number indicated. Turn to that page and do the exercise with your book next to you so that you can check the instructions and illustrations frequently. Then turn back to the *Routines* section and do the next exercise or procedure. Do the Week One Routine of Exercise, Breathing, and Meditation every day of the first week as your **Main Routine.** Then go on to Week Two.

WEEK ONE

EXERCISE	BREATHING	MEDITATION	NUTRITION	PHILOSOPHY
Begin with some simple chair exercises after reading page 32. * **Shoulder Shrugs** p. 33 * **Single & Double Arm Reaches** p. 37 * **Elbow Rolls** p. 34 * **Seated Leg Lift** p. 41 * **Seated Knee Squeezes** p. 41 * **Folded Pose (first part)** p. 38 * **Tip Toe Breath** p. 45 * **Standing Reach** p. 43	First read Section 7, Breathing. * **Belly Breath** p. 83 Do 1 minute of Belly Breath before any of your other exercises. Then do your exercise routine after which you should do 3 more minutes of Belly Breath. You will also do 3–5 minutes of Belly Breath this week in your Mini Routine.	After doing your exercise and breathing, **turn to your Complete Relaxation Procedure on page 89.** Do this for about 10 minutes, followed by 10–15 minutes of the OM Meditation technique. **NOTE: If you are unaccustomed to being on the floor, do your relaxation and meditation on your bed. Remember to not be disturbed by family, friends, your pets, or the phone during meditation.**	This first week you should thoroughly read and review the nutrition section. You should try to understand the difference between **under-nutrition and over-nutrition (page 101)**, as well as the various nutrition hints found in the **"What You Can Do To Help Yourself"** section on pages 102–104. 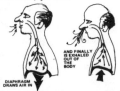	This first week you should read the entire philosophy section and **study the "5 Ways To Increase Personal Growth" on page 111.** Go to your library or bookstore and pick up a copy of *Transformations* (see the reading list, page 111). Begin to read and study this book on personality transformations.

WEEK TWO

EXERCISE	BREATHING	MEDITATION	NUTRITION	PHILOSOPHY
Continue with the exercises from Week One and add a few. * **Shoulder Shrugs** p. 33 * **Single & Double Arm Reaches** p. 37 * **Elbow Rolls** p. 34 * **Elbow & Shoulder To Knee** p. 39 * **Seated Leg Lift** p. 41 * **Seated Knee Squeezes** p. 41 * **Folded Pose (add Folded Rest)** p. 38 * **Tip Toe Breath** p. 45 * **Standing Reach** p. 43 * **Standing Leg Lifts** p. 46	* **Belly Breath** p. 83 Do 1 minute of Belly Breath before beginning your exercise routine, and try it against the wall. After doing your exercise routine, do another session of Belly Breath for 2 minutes, and then **try 2 or 3 minutes of Complete Breath, p. 84.** 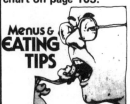 AND FINALLY IS EXHALED OUT OF THE BODY DIAPHRAGM DRAWS AIR IN	After doing your exercise and breathing, complete your Main Routine with 5–10 minutes of Complete Relaxation **followed by 10–15 minutes of Silent Awareness Training (SAT). This week you'll do 10–15 minutes of SAT rather than OM Meditation.** Remember: this exercise, breathing, and meditation routine is your Main Routine. Don't forget to do your Mini Routine also.	This **week make a concerted attempt to incorporate some of the 7 Ways To Eat Less Bad Food and More Good Food.** To help yourself, **make a list of everything you eat this week.** Write it all down, and at the end of the week **review it against the chart on page 105.** Menus & **EATING TIPS**	This week make it a point to **form a study group with a few of your friends.** Set up a schedule for your group to meet once a week or every few days and decide which books and topics you will discuss for the next month. Remember: stay away from idle gossip and keep to your lofty topic. If you have already finished *Transformations*, choose another book on the reading list to explore.

WEEK THREE

EXERCISE	BREATHING	MEDITATION	NUTRITION	PHILOSOPHY
As you notice, we are going to slowly increase the number of exercises you do each day. * Shoulder Shrugs p. 33 * Arm Reaches p. 37 * Elbow Rolls p. 34 * Elbow & Shoulder To Knee p. 39 * Head Rotations p. 36 * Arm Rotations p. 38 * Seated Leg Lift p. 41 * Seated Knee Squeezes p. 41 * Folded Pose p. 38 * Tip Toe Breath p. 45 * Standing Reach p. 43 * Standing Leg Lifts p. 46 * Gentle Full Bends p. 49	* Do 1 minute of Belly Breath followed by 2 minutes of Complete Breath before exercising. * Then after your exercises, do 3—5 minutes of Complete Breath before your Relaxation/ Meditation Period. * Add 3—5 minutes of Complete Breath to your Mini Routine. * Try Relaxing Breath in bed this week.	After the exercise and breathing portions of your Main Routine, finish with 10—20 minutes of Relaxation & Meditation. **Remember: this week choose whichever meditation you find the easiest: either OM Meditation or SAT. For the next 3 months practice only one of the techniques after your Complete Relaxation procedure.** 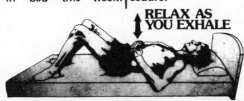 **RELAX AS YOU EXHALE**	Go to the library or bookstore and begin to read and study about nutrition. Three of the best books we can recommend are: **Let's Eat Right to Keep Fit,** Adelle Davis, B.A., Harcourt, Brace & Co., N.Y. 1954. **Diet For a Small Planet,** Frances Moore Lappe, Ballantine Books, Inc., N.Y. 1971. **Composition of Foods,** Bernice K. Watt & Annabel L. Merrill, U.S. Dept. of Agriculture, 1963.	**This week make a concerted effort to live in the present.** Stop yourself from talking and thinking about the past and focus your conversation and thinking on the present. Make a list of weekly or daily personal goals and set up step-by-step plans to achieve those goals. This will help you to think more about today and less about yesterday or tomorrow.

WEEK FOUR

EXERCISE	BREATHING	MEDITATION	NUTRITION	PHILOSOPHY
This week we want you to try some floor exercises along with your other exercises. So do all of the chair exercises that you did in Week Three, and then **turn directly to page 50 and practice getting up and down on the floor using a chair.** Once you're down on the floor, do the following: * Gentle Twist p. 52 * Foot Flap p. 52	* Do 2—3 minutes of Complete Breath before beginning your exercises. * Then after your exercises, remain on the floor and do the **Relaxing Breath (page 86) before your Meditation Period.** * **For your Mini Routine you should try the Humming Breath (page 85) for 2—5 minutes followed by 10--15 minutes of Seated Meditation. See page 94.**	You have now been practicing your meditation for 3 weeks or so, and hopefully you have now chosen one of the two meditation techniques to practice every day after your Complete Relaxation. **It's now time to try the Seated Meditation (page 94), so put that into your Mini Routine at another time of the day.**	This week continue to apply the 7 Ways to Eat Less Bad Food and More Good Food, and try to incorporate some of the Eating Tips on page 106 into your menu. Don't forget, if you have constipation, see page 106; and **above all, start reading the labels on your packaged foods. Eat food, not chemicals.**	Encourage your study group to invite some new members to attend your meetings. If you look, you can find many willing young people, clergymen, teachers, psychologists, or other interesting people to give your group some new insights and unfamiliar directions. **Remember to talk about your own ideas, and not just what you've read, to improve your ability to say what you mean and to hear what others have to say about what you think.**

Don't forget to massage your muscles & joints during or after your exercises - pp. 75, 76.
Rest frequently between exercises.

WEEK FIVE

EXERCISE	BREATHING	MEDITATION	NUTRITION	PHILOSOPHY
This week you should concentrate a little more on improving your floor exercises. * Shoulder Shrugs p. 33 * Arm Reaches p. 37 * Elbow Rolls p. 34 * Seated Leg Lifts p. 41 * Knee Squeezes p. 41 * Standing Rear Leg Lifts p. 47 * Getting Up & Down pp. 50–51 * Gentle Twist p. 52 * Knee Squeezes p. 53 * Easy Sit-Up p. 55 * Spine Twist p. 58 * Easy Cobra Lift p. 60	Now that you've been practicing for 4 or 5 weeks, your daily routine should be getting well established. Example: * First thing in the morning (in bed or seated on the edge), 2–5 minutes of either Belly Breath, Complete Breath, Humming Breath, or Relaxing Breath. * Main Routine: before exercising—2 minutes Complete Breath; after exercising—5 minutes Complete Breath. * Mini Routine: 5 minutes Complete Breath before meditation.	Your meditation schedule should also be getting well established. Example: * Main Routine: after exercising and breathing, do 5–10 minutes of Complete Relaxation followed by 10–15 minutes of either OM Meditation or SAT. * Mini Routine: after doing 5 minutes of breathing, do 10 minutes of Complete Relaxation followed by 10–15 minutes of meditation. Remember, your Mini Routine is done at a different time of day than your Main Routine.	Note Harry and Clara Harvey's suggestion on page 105 for losing weight. If you can cut down on sugar and sweet desserts, you will probably drastically cut your daily calorie intake and may also lose weight. Substitute fresh fruits and juices for soda pop and candy, and most importantly, stop buying junk food. If you can control your sweet tooth in the grocery store, it will be a lot easier to eat a piece of fruit for that midnight snack because you won't have junk food within reach.	This week you should put some piece of wisdom or an ethical or moral principle to the test in your daily life. Try it in real-life situations, and force yourself to examine its effect on you, on others, and on the situation you are applying it to. Do concepts such as truthfulness, nonviolence, humility, or compassion have any real practical application? Talk about your experiences with others and find out what they think. Be open to new ideas.

WEEK SIX

EXERCISE	BREATHING	MEDITATION	NUTRITION	PHILOSOPHY
By now you should be doing exercises from all three sections. Do all Chair Exercises on pages 33–42. Standing Exercises: * Standing Reaches p. 43 * Tip Toe Breath p. 45 * Leg Lifts pp. 46–47 * Gentle Full Bends p. 49 Floor Exercises: * Getting Up & Down pp. 50–51 * Gentle Twist & Foot Flap p. 52 * Knee Squeezes p. 53 * Easy Sit-Up p. 55 * Seated Sun Pose p. 56 * Spine Twist p. 58 * Easy Cobra p. 60 * All Fours Leg Lift p. 63 * Baby Pose p. 66	You now do some breathing in the morning during your Main Routine, and again in your Mini Routine. You should now be practicing about 5–10 minutes of Complete Breath in your Main Routine and 5 minutes in your Mini Routine, plus maybe some Relaxing Breath in bed. You might now begin to try the Stomach Lift on page 86. It is a superb exercise for breathing and health.	For total fitness, the mind needs both exercise and proper rest, so meditate regularly. Try to follow your Main and Mini Routines with the prescribed amount of meditation and relaxation. You should also be trying the seated meditation position. Try to relax more and more into silence, and if you're doing the OM Meditation, try to center and focus your mind on OM so that there are fewer distractions.	This week get in the habit of asking yourself: "Why am I eating this?" before you put anything in your mouth. Ask yourself, "Am I eating this because I really want it, or because I'm just used to eating this food at this time?" Look at your plate before you start to eat, and ask yourself how you could make your meal more nutritious. Remind yourself at every meal that eating better makes you feel better!	If you have followed the routines for the past five weeks, you probably have a good feeling for the type of intellectual, spiritual, and philosophical challenge that we are encouraging. Now keep up the good work! Maybe you have decided to go back to school or become more active in the religious or theological (not just social!) functions in your church, temple, or community. Expand your frontiers to other unfamiliar philosophical ground in your study groups and make the pursuit of wisdom a regular part of every day!

YOUR DAILY BASICS
Every day~10 to 20 min. Exercise
5 to 15 min. Breathing
20 to 40 min. Meditation

DIET & NUTRITION SECTION 10

"I can't afford what I eat now I'm just too old and fat to care, and besides, I may die tomorrow!"

MILLIONS OF ELDERLY SUFFER FROM
MALNUTRITION

Older people frequently get defensive when the subject of nutrition is brought up and try to hide the fact that they know they should improve their diet. Most people think that the term malnutrition means starvation or getting too little food. But actually, it has two definitions:

OVERNUTRITION: eating too much of the wrong foods. UNDERNUTRITION: eating too little of the right foods. Older people in our country suffer from both sides of the malnutrition problem.

OVER NUTRITION

The average American eats over 100 pounds of plain sugar each year and more than double that amount of high-saturated fat meats and meat products. Most of us eat too many high-phosphorus, low-calcium meats instead of eggs, dairy products, and vegetable-protein foods. Chances are that your diet is simply too rich for your own good.

Eating too much sugar, all types of fat, calories, salt, cholesterol, alcohol, and phosphorus are major causes of:

**Cancer,
Strokes, Obesity,
Diabetes, Arthritis, Heart Disease,
High Blood Pressure, Osteoporosis,
Cirrhosis of the Liver,
Hardening of the Arteries.**

UNDER NUTRITION

Surveys of older people's diets have revealed that the average person over 65 eats far less of the high-quality foods, such as dairy products, eggs, fresh fruits and vegetables, and whole-grain bread products, than is needed for good health.

As a result of poor eating habits, low income, and many other interrelated factors, the following nutrients are commonly undersupplied in the older person's diet:

**Iron, Vitamin B-Complex,
Calcium, Vitamin C,
Vitamin A, Protein.**

This undernutrition causes:
**Depression, Anemia, Rapid Aging,
Excessive Fatigue, Weak, Easily Broken Bones,
Low Infection Resistance,
Gum Disease and Loss of Teeth.**

WHAT YOU CAN DO TO HELP YOURSELF

Proper nutrition keeps us free from disease by bolstering the defenses of the body and by providing the right balance of protein, fat, and carbohydrates. This keeps arteries and blood free from fats, maintains normal weight, and protects the vital organs from degeneration. Here are some specific diet-disease relationships and some suggestions on how to avoid these problems. IT IS VITAL THAT YOU ALWAYS GET QUALIFIED MEDICAL TREATMENT FOR ANY OF THESE PROBLEMS.

Obesity

Obesity is the largest health problem of old age. Triggered by inactivity, it shortens your life and increases your chances of having a heart attack or stroke and of developing arthritis, diabetes, or cancer. Obesity in the poor, the black, and other minority groups is double or triple the rate in other older groups.

What you should do

Eat less sugar, fats and oils, and use low-fat or skim-milk dairy products. This means avoiding candy, pastry, pie, and cakes, and broiling or baking instead of frying. Eat as many fresh fruits and vegetables as you like (served without rich sauces or too much butter or margarine), dark green, leafy vegetables, and salad vegetables. Limit or cut out alcohol entirely, and replace all soft drinks with club soda over ice, with a wedge of lemon. Exercise is absolutely essential. Do your Easy Does It Yoga program every day for the strength and stability you need to lose all that excess flab!

Cancer

Cancer Cancer kills many thousands of Americans yearly. Those who eat a lot of meat fat and sugar, who use tobacco, and who are heavy drinkers, have far more cancer than those who do not. Deficiencies of vitamins A, C, and E increase cancer risk, as do too little fiber and deficiencies of the trace mineral selenium.

What you should do

Meat, especially beef, is the primary source of fat in your diet. If you must eat meat, trim off all visible fat, drain off all fat during cooking, never eat meat gravy or processed meats. Never use meat fat for cooking, and cut back drastically on fried foods. Replace whole milk and high-fat dairy foods with skim or low-fat milk and cheeses. Eat more fresh fruits and vegetables and whole-grain breads and cereals; they supply fiber, vitamins A, C, and E, and selenium. Stop using tobacco, get rid of excess fat on your body, and reduce alcohol to under five drinks weekly.

OVER PROCESSED FOODS
SUGAR
ARTIFICIAL COLOR
ARTIFICIAL FLAVOR
BHA
BHT
HIGH CO$T LOW INCOME

Heart Attacks, Strokes, Hardening of Arteries, & High Blood Pressure

The typical American diet is causing a virtual epidemic of heart and artery diseases by building up fats in the bloodstream and causing high blood pressure. As fats accumulate in the bloodstream, they block circulation, resulting in coronary artery disease, strokes, high blood pressure, hardening of the arteries, memory loss, headaches, dizziness, cold hands and feet, stasis ulcers, gangrene, and poor healing of cuts and broken bones. Excessive salt intake, a characteristic of our diet, also raises blood pressure.

What you should do.

Get rid of excessive weight. Stop using tobacco completely and do your Easy Does It Yoga and other exercises every day. Substitute high-quality, low-fat protein foods such as eggs, cottage cheese, buttermilk, and nutritional yeast for saturated fat foods such as processed meats, beef, and pork. Limit both butter and margarine, and eat more high-fiber fresh fruits and vegetables. Vitamins A, C, and E help keep your circulatory system healthy, and two or three tablespoons of fresh, granular lecithin on cereal or in soups help reduce blood fats.

Diabetes

Diabetes is caused by a deficiency of a hormone—insulin—which brings sugar from the blood into the cells. Diabetics need either to replace insulin with shots and oral doses, or to reduce the need for insulin with strict diets. If possible, diet management without supplemental insulin is more desirable, causing fewer heart and artery complications. Some nutritionists believe that a diet high in magnesium, B-complex vitamins, vitamin C, and the trace mineral chromium can reduce insulin needs or restore your own insulin production. Chromium is needed for insulin's effectiveness, and this deficiency may account for many prediabetic conditions.

What you should do.

First, you must lose excess weight. Eat small, frequent, well-balanced meals, Important foods to include are eggs, low-fat dairy foods, fresh fruits and vegetables, dried peas and beans, and whole-grain breads and cereals. Be sure to make any changes in your diet within the framework of your prescribed diabetic diet. Drink nutritional yeast before every meal to get high amounts of B vitamins. Nutritional yeast is also the richest source of chromium. Three to five grams of vitamin C and 400-800 I.U. of vitamin E are also helpful. Three tablespoons of granular lecithin and the magnesium of seven dolomite tablets daily will help remove fats from the blood and reduce complications.

Arthritis

Many experts feel arthritis is a stress disease in which connective tissue in the joints becomes painfully inflamed. Stiffness and calicfcation result if the disease is not reversed.

What you should do.

Get rid of excess fat, and then meet the increased nutritional requirements of stress with a diet high in B vitamins (particularly pantothenic acid) and vitamin C. Begin each meal with a glass of nutritional yeast. Eat plenty of low-fat protein from eggs, dairy products, and dried peas and beans. Extra vitamin E and the calcium and magnesium from dolomite help to prevent stiffening and calcification. One or two tablespoons daily of vegetable oils from mayonnaise, salad dressing, or nuts help hormone production which is important in keeping painful swelling in check. Above all, remember that nutritional yeast is the best antistress food available, and extra vitamins C and E and dolomite help to prevent or relieve some of the discomfort of arthritis.

Constipation

Older people are bombarded by advertisements to convince them that they need a laxative for a daily bowel movement. Laxatives can be addictive and harmful to your health. The primary cause of constipation is that fiber and roughage have been almost completely removed from our diet. Lack of fiber has also been implicated in adding to other problems such as colitis, diverticulitis, and intestinal cancer.

What you should do.

Drink 4-6 eight-ounce glasses of nutritious fluids daily. Eat only whole-grain breads and cereals, fresh fruits, and fresh vegetables. Adding extra wheat bran to your diet may also be helpful. Exercise is essential. See page 20 for exercises that relieve constipation. If you follow these nutritional hints and exercise daily, you may try not using laxatives. FOR ACID INDIGESTION. Instead of an antacid preparation, try drinking a big glass of buttermilk or nutritional yeast. The protein will neutralize the acids in your stomach and give you a big nutritonal boost as well.

Osteoporosis

This disease is characterized by weak, brittle bones. It can affect the jaw bone and cause teeth to be lost due to gum disease. These problems are caused in part by too little calcium and fluoride and too much high-phosphorus food, particularly meat.

What you should do.

Replace meat with low-fat dairy products and eggs. These supply calcium and vitamin D. Drink fluoridated water, and eat whole grains, nuts, and dark green, leafy vegetables, which supply zinc and magnesium. If you already have osteoporosis, take dolomite for extra calcium and magnesium.

Confusion, Poor Appetite, Melancholy, & Listlessness

These are symptoms that may or may not be accompanied by aches and pains; nonetheless, they are very upsetting.

What you should do.

No one knows the specific cause of these complaints, but we do know that you can help yourself get rid of these symptoms by eating better. We feel that the most important thing that you can do for these problems is add B-complex vitamins to your diet from nutritional yeast. Remember that the B vitamins are a team, and you must be sure to get some of all of them.

Muscle Cramps, Restless Legs, Anxiety, & Insomnia
When the arteries are blocked with fats, blood-carrying oxygen and calcium can't reach the muscles in the legs and feet. Cramps then result when you exercise the muscles or when the blood pressure drops at night.

What you should do.

You need vitamin E supplements to increase circulation, and calcium and magnesium from dolomite tablets to boost muscle tissue concentrations. Try 600 I.U. vitamin E daily for six months to a year, and try three dolomite tablets before each meal. Also increase dairy products and dark green, leafy vegetables.

Nutritional Anemia
Pallor, depression, and lack of energy and stamina are symptoms of iron deficiency, one of several causes of anemia. Folate deficiency anemia is common where there are no fresh fruits and vegetables in the diet. Deficiencies of vitamins B-6 or E, or magnesium can also cause anemia, as can deficiencies of folic acid and vitamin C.

What you should do.

Eat plenty of unrefined foods which are rich in iron, particularly blackstrap molasses, wheat germ, green leafy vegetables, dried fruits, and whole-grain breads and cereals. Fresh fruits and vegetables high in folic acid and vitamin C with foods high in vitamin E and magnesium are also necessary.

FOR A LONG HEALTHY LIFE...

The new science of nutrition has uncovered a direct relationship between malnutrition and illness. The illnesses caused by malnutrition shorten life and make our later years dreadful. Scientists have concrete suggestions to help us live longer.

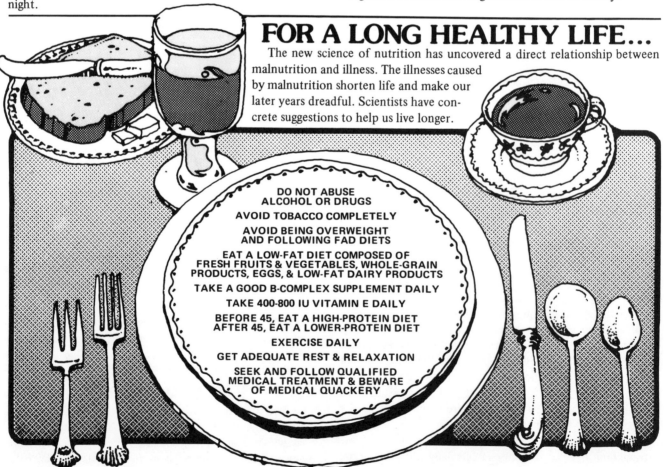

DO NOT ABUSE
ALCOHOL OR DRUGS

AVOID TOBACCO COMPLETELY

AVOID BEING OVERWEIGHT
AND FOLLOWING FAD DIETS

EAT A LOW-FAT DIET COMPOSED OF
FRESH FRUITS & VEGETABLES, WHOLE-GRAIN
PRODUCTS, EGGS, & LOW-FAT DAIRY PRODUCTS

TAKE A GOOD B-COMPLEX SUPPLEMENT DAILY

TAKE 400-800 IU VITAMIN E DAILY

BEFORE 45, EAT A HIGH-PROTEIN DIET
AFTER 45, EAT A LOWER-PROTEIN DIET

EXERCISE DAILY

GET ADEQUATE REST & RELAXATION

SEEK AND FOLLOW QUALIFIED
MEDICAL TREATMENT & BEWARE
OF MEDICAL QUACKERY

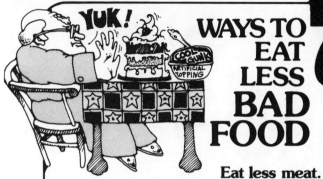

7 WAYS TO EAT LESS BAD FOOD | 7 WAYS TO EAT MORE GOOD FOOD

WAYS TO EAT LESS BAD FOOD		WAYS TO EAT MORE GOOD FOOD
Eat less meat.	1	Eat high-protein, low-fat dairy foods.
Use less frozen and canned convenience foods.	2	Eat plenty of fresh fruits and vegetables.
Don't eat white bread.	3	Eat only whole-grain breads.
Don't eat lard, meat fat, or margarine.	4	Eat one or two tablespoons of vegetable oil daily.
Eat as little sugar as possible.	5	Eat unsugared fresh fruits and fruit salads for dessert.
Eat less at night when you're inactive.	6	Eat more during the day when you're active.
Avoid artificial "chemical" foods.	7	Buy food, not chemicals. Read the labels.

EAT LESS

PROCESSED MEATS bacon / hot dogs / sausage / fatback / cold cuts
REFINED FOODS white breads / pasta / refined cereals / white rice
SATURATED FATS lard / meat fat / butter
SWEETS cake / sweet rolls / candy / pastry
CHEMICAL FOODS margarine / nondairy creamers / nondairy dessert toppings / imitation juices / diet soda pop / artificially flavored and colored foods and desserts
STIMULANTS coffee / tea

EAT MORE

LOW-FAT DAIRY skim milk / cottage cheese / yogurt / buttermilk / eggs
ROUGHAGE apples / broccoli / Brussels sprouts / wheat bran / greens / raw carrots
GREENS spinach / kale / mustard greens / turnip greens
FRESH FRUITS & FRUIT JUICES
NUTS / WHOLE-GRAIN BREADS & CEREALS
A LITTLE VEGETABLE OIL mayonnaise / salad dressing
DRIED PEAS & BEANS
NUTRITIONAL YEAST

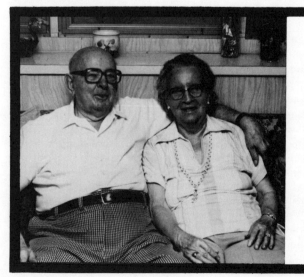

"The doctor said Harry's blood sugar was too high, so we decided that we'd go without sugar. We made a study of it by reading the labels. You'd be surprised how many things have sugar in them, and a lot of it! One thing I watch most of all is the cereal. We could only find two that don't contain sugar. I make sure that everything we eat doesn't have sugar in it. And do you know what's happened? Harry's blood sugar level went right back down where it should be, and **we lost weight fast!** We didn't intend to lose weight, we just did it for our health. **It is surely the easiest way to lose weight that there is!**"

Alice Christensen's parents, **Harry & Clara Harvey**
84 & 82 / Venice, Florida

Breakfast

1. Your first meal of the day should give you energy and protein to last most of the day. Begin each meal with at least one teaspoon of nutritional yeast stirred into a glass of fruit juice.

2. COTTAGE CHEESE & YOGURT with fresh fruit.

3. UNSWEETENED FRUIT JUICE.

4. One or more of the following:
* whole-wheat or bran toast with one teaspoon of butter.
* oatmeal or other whole-grain cereals such as Ralston, Maypo, or Wheatena, cooked with skim milk, not water, and flavored with fruit, a little dark brown sugar or honey, and raisins, nuts, or sunflower seeds.
* soft-boiled, poached, or scrambled eggs (limit: 4—6 eggs weekly).
* hard cheese and tomato broiled on whole-wheat toast.
* Grapenuts, Shredded Wheat, All Bran, or other whole-grain, cold cereal without added sugar, served with skim milk, and sweetened with sliced banana and raisins. *[Not granolas, because they usually have a very high sugar content.]*
* whole-wheat or buckwheat pancakes with stewed fruit such as applesauce.
* wheat germ, an excellent source of iron and B-complex vitamins, can be added to pancake mixes or added liberally to cottage cheese, yogurt, and cereal.

5. GLASS OF BUTTERMILK.

Lunch

1. NUTRITIONAL YEAST DRINK (see breakfast).

2. One of the following:
* open-faced broiled sandwich with cheese, lots of vegetables, and a fresh fruit salad.
* big, fresh, green salad with grated cheese, vegetables, olives, oil-and-vinegar dressing, served with bran muffins.
* hearty vegetable soup made with brown rice and red kidney beans, served with whole-wheat crackers and cheese.
* noodle casserole (whole wheat is best) cooked with cream of mushroom soup and some vegetable and cheese. *[Can be made ahead of time, frozen in aluminum pie plates, and heated in the oven.]*
* a steamed vegetable such as broccoli, cauliflower, Brussels sprouts , or greens, broiled with cheese and bread crumbs, with delicious broiled tomatoes.

Avoid Constipation

To avoid constipation, every day eat:

2 TABLESPOONS WHEAT BRAN
1 SERVING OF GREEN SALAD
1 PIECE OF HARD FRUIT
SEVERAL GLASSES OF WATER

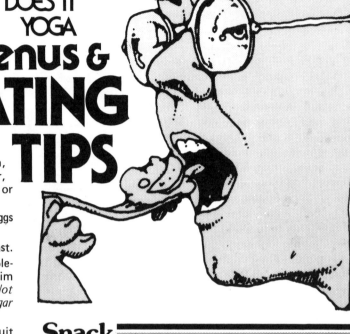

EASY DOES IT YOGA
Menus & EATING TIPS

Snack

1. GLASS OF BUTTERMILK

2. One of the following:
* roasted soy beans, sunflower seeds, and nuts.
* peanut butter without additives on whole-wheat bread, whole-wheat crackers, or celery.
* you can eat all you want of raw carrots, celery, and other vegetables and fresh fruits such as apples, oranges, bananas, avocados, and grapefruits.

Supper

1. NUTRITIONAL YEAST DRINK (see breakfast).

2. One of the following:
* succotash made with lima beans, whole-kernel corn, and red pimentos.
* mixed vegetable or creamed soup with broiled cheese and tomato open-face sandwich.
* large fresh fruit salad with yogurt dressing and whole-wheat crackers.
* three-bean salad made with kidney beans and Italian dressing, served with cheese toast.
* broiled mustard or turnip greens sauteed in oil, onions, garlic and spices, with cottage cheese on the side.
* cook one package of brown rice every week and keep it in a tightly closed container in the refrigerator. Use it with vegetable stew, boiled beans, greens, and soups throughout the week.
* cold cereal with cottage cheese and fresh fruit.
* spinach salad with cottage cheese and broiled grapefruit.
* a broiled open-faced cheese sandwich and fresh coleslaw.

EASY DOES IT YOGA
NUTRITION GLOSSARY

Vitamin A prevents infection and tumors, maintains acute vision, and keeps the skin beautiful. TO INCREASE VITAMIN A you should eat more dairy products and deeply colored fruits and vegetables. [Toxic at high doses.]

Vitamin B-Complex prevents widespread symptoms ranging from anemia, poor posture, indigestion and depression to neuritis. TO INCREASE B-COMPLEX VITAMINS you should eat more nutritional yeast, whole grains, nuts and seeds. Yogurt, buttermilk, and cottage cheese establish bacteria in your intestines which produce B vitamins.

Vitamin C repairs bones, cartilage, discs, and blood vessels. It breaks up blood fats, increases the antiarthritic hormones, and kills harmful bacteria and viruses. TO INCREASE VITAMIN C, you should eat more dark green vegetables and citrus fruits. Ascorbic acid tablets and powder are cheap and effective too.

Vitamin D controls the mineral metabolism of the bones. TO INCREASE VITAMIN D you should eat more dairy foods and supplemented cereal foods. One-fourth stick of butter contains 30 IU of vitamin D, and one cup of enriched milk contains 100 IU. Under certain conditions it is produced on the skin by sunshine. [Toxic at high doses.]

Vitamin E regulates aging by controlling oxidation of enzymes, fatty structures, and hormones. It also prevents unwanted blood clots and reduces muscle cramps and "restless legs." TO INCREASE VITAMIN E you should eat more nuts, seeds, and wheat germ. Vitamin E supplements are widely sold and are not expensive.

Calcium & Magnesium are natural tranquilizers and keep the bones and teeth strong. TO INCREASE CALCIUM & MAGNESIUM, you should eat more dairy foods, dark green, leafy vegetables, nuts, whole grains, and dolomite, a deep-mined mineral available in tablets.

Iron prevents an anemia which can be recognized by pallor, shortness of breath, brittle nails, heart palpitations, forgetfulness, and depression. TO INCREASE IRON you should eat blackstrap molasses, nutritional yeast, wheat germ, and wheat bran.

Iodine increases your energy and boosts circulation. TO INCREASE IODINE you should use only iodized salt.

Chromium increases glucose tolerance. TO INCREASE CHROMIUM you should eat more nutritional yeast and whole-grain products.

Fluoride forms strong bones and teeth. TO INCREASE FLUORIDE, drink fluoridated water.

Nutritional Yeast is the best source of all the B-complex vitamin team. Add it to your diet slowly, starting with one teaspoonful in unsweetened fruit juice or water before a meal, like a cocktail. Slowly increase this amount to one tablespoon, three times a day. Ask your druggist or grocer to order brewer's yeast of primary type in *powder* form. Flakes or chips are more expensive and less potent.

Lecithin an extract of soybeans, is an emulsifier of blood fats. It helps prevent the cholesterol deposits that cause hardening of the arteries. The B vitamins in it also help protect the liver from cirrhosis. Granular lecithin can also be obtained from your druggist or grocer. Keep it refrigerated. You might add it to blender drinks, put it on cereal or in soups, or just stir it into your yeast cocktail.

Fresh Fruits & Vegetables should be washed immediately in cold water, dried thoroughly, and put in the refrigerator or other cold, dark place. Serve them raw, directly from the refrigerator, or cooked by rapid steaming in inexpensive vegetable steamers available from most stores. This waterless method preserves the flavor, color, and nutritional content of your food. If possible, do not peel vegetables, or instead, peel them *after* cooking, just before serving.

Low-Fat Protein keeps fat out of your arteries and helps you to lose weight safely. Found in eggs, low-fat dairy products, and combinations of peas and beans with grains such as whole-wheat, oatmeal, and brown rice. It is also cheaper and easier to digest than the high-fat protein from meat. Eggs contain cholesterol, it is true, but we now know that saturated fat, which eggs are free of, is the thing to avoid.

EASY DOES IT YOGA PHILOSOPHY
SECTION 11

"Young man... all is constantly changing. I am housed in my real Self, which does not change, unlike my body, which will grow old and die. Maybe as you grow older, you will understand this point more clearly." SWAMI RAMA (1900-1972)

BY ALICE CHRISTENSEN

The goal of Yoga is to give you a philosophic outlook which enables you to understand yourself and to find lasting beauty and happiness in yourself, in others, and in the world around you. The great scholar of Yoga, Patanjali, taught that as we become more and more quiet, we learn more about ourselves, our thoughts, and our feelings. As self-control and inner quiet develop, an intensely pleasurable experience of strength and clarity of consciousness begins to grow. When you become really quiet, you are able to see the real you and discover that there is a lot more in each of us than meets the eye.

In looking at the way my own life and perspectives have changed over the years, one of the clearest memories I have is that of my teacher Rama. He had just come to this country. Though 62 years old when we first met, I can still remember his golden complexion, unforgettable eyes, and his tremendous strength and vitality. Despite his age he could outthink and even outrun me. He was a powerful testimony to the value of Yoga for older people. He recognized our country's tragic tendency to discard people as they grow old, and he was the finest example to me that this pathetic waste did not have to be.

That was Rama. Although he died here in Cleveland, Ohio, in 1972, he remains a constant inspiration for all of us. What he taught me and represented in himself by a beautiful example was that my typical American outlook on death was impractical and wasteful. Rama taught me that your later years are the sum and substance of how you live when

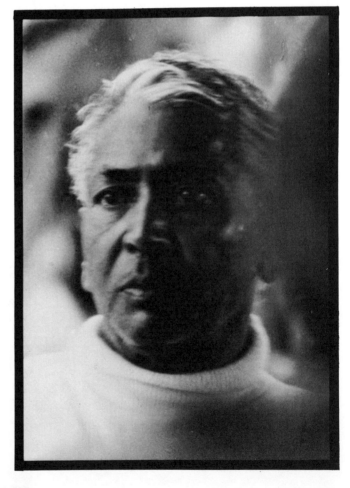

you are young. Virtue and morality then have meaning, because these disciplines give you solace and satisfaction as you get older. I learned from Rama that my life, my body, and my mind were created to grow and mature in wisdom throughout my entire life. Through my practice of Yoga I was able to utilize these new ideas and become more aware of my inner self. I studied all the philosophy I could get my hands on, trying to see the various perspectives on life and death. I was particularly touched by the *Bhagavad-Gita*, which describes the inner self: "As a man discarding worn-out clothes takes others which are new, likewise the embodied soul, casting off worn-out bodies, enters into others which are new. Weapons cannot cut it, nor can fire burn it, water cannot drench it, nor can wind make it dry."

It was not until I had an experience in meditation of slipping out of my body that I really saw the truth of what Rama had said to me. I suddenly found myself looking down at my body. It was still there, on the floor, but I was looking at it from high above. I knew then that no matter how dear my limited concept of myself was to me, it was not the total picture at all.

"Nothing is permanent, even the body I am living in is not permanent. Time will change all of this. Even the mountains around us will rise and fall."

As one gains in years, it is essential that the mind begin to delve into the more subtle, abstract issues and concepts of both life and death to discover what is lasting and real about ourselves. The appropriate product of retirement years is not physical, but mental and philosophical. We are so geared to thinking in terms of products that we have forgotten that you can't put wisdom in a box and set it on the table. It must be lived, experienced, and transmitted. This product-orientation of our culture has enslaved our people to an image of the robot-like company man who is only a small part of a vast machine which spews out endless items for consumption in the material world. This forced conformity into identical production machines is a bloodletting of our creativity. Real self-awareness, which Yoga enhances, consistently offers new creative patterns to help us live better and happier lives. This materialistic concept has become so engrained in our society that the physical outer world has become overvalued. You must see its worth, but balance it with a mature outlook which recognizes the value of intangibles.

A simple story about Rama illustrates the transient nature of our physical world. *Rama had a friend who owned a small piece of land on the banks of the Ganges, between the cities of Haridwar and Rishikesh, in northern India. Rama liked the atmosphere of this place very much, and since the man had no use for the land, he gave it to Rama. After a year or so, I was visiting him there for advanced training in Yoga, and the hut in which he lived had been converted into two or three rooms with cement walls and a tin roof. Rama didn't realize that permanent structures on the flood side of the dike were prohibited by an obscure ruling in the municipal codes of Haridwar.*

One Sunday, a zealous young official came into the compound and approached Rama. "Respected sir, I must tell you that your building here is in violation of the Permanent Structure Code."

Rama replied, "What permanent structure?"

The young man walked over to the kitchen wall and kicked it as he said, "What do you mean—is this not meant

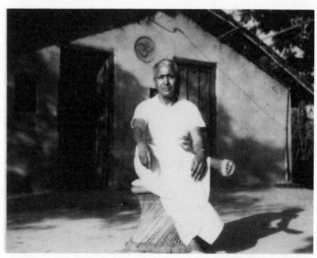

to be a permanent structure?"

Rama calmly replied, "Young man, even those large temples on the city side of the dike may seem permanent to you. However, nothing is permanent. Even the body that I am living in is not permanent. Time will change all of this. Even the mountains around us will rise and fall. Your kicking of an impermanent structure with your impermanent body and calling it permanent makes little sense to me. All is constantly changing. I am housed in my real Self, which does not change, unlike my body, which will grow old and die. Maybe as you get older, you will understand this point more clearly."

Although the legal issues were unresolved, the official realized that he was dealing with a philosophical code which was more binding than the city regulations. He paid Rama his respects and let the matter rest.

The fearless attitude of my teacher, coupled with his insight into the deeper issues of existence helped me gain the most precious thing in my life: I no longer fear the loss of my body in death. I have experienced a change of heart, and my life has taken a new direction because of him. I am more compassionate towards my body and others in this world. I feel that now is the time to present these ageless concepts which can help people everywhere use their bodies and minds effectively to pass through the difficult door to wisdom that lies in the later years of one's life. We have designed a program which supports you during this difficult transition to an active, independent life. The Easy Does It Yoga system gives you the tools to help yourself govern your own later years.

The ideal age to begin to practice is traditionally 53. Yogis believe that the best time for self-growth and reflection is after the passions of youth have subsided, families are grown, and our debt to society has been paid. In this new stage of life, your primary responsibility is to improve yourself. Only by fulfilling this responsibility to yourself can you provide an effective role model for the younger generation to emulate and provide a vital counterbalance to the younger elements of society. Age can then be a great source of leadership which is needed not only in this country, but in the entire world.

Yoga means union, or to join together, as with a yoke. The main product of Yoga is to end separateness not only within one's own self but with society and the world as well. The lack of separateness produces a person who is truly whole, able to face life well fortified with strength and balanced judgment.

Patanjali's *Yoga Sutras,* one of the earliest written records of Yoga practice, defines Yoga as "the control of the thought waves of the mind." This increased mental control is a powerful agent which helps to alleviate unshakable feelings of depression, anger, and fear. These emotional upsets become the subject of the conversation which goes on in your mind incessantly. This conversation feeds and prolongs the emotional upset and saps your energy as well. The pattern of this destructive cycle can be broken by the detachment given you by the philosophy of Yoga which says that you are more than only a body with feelings and a mind. Yoga gives you a higher perspective that allows you to see that most thoughts and feelings have no real basis. They seem to be more powerful than they really are. Easy Does It Yoga meditation also helps to break up these cycles of emotional upset by creating a daily habit of a quiet mental vacation which rests the mind. When you return to your everyday concerns, you get a new look at the mind's reactions to them, which gives you a fresh, possibly more effective, approach to your problems.

Yoga teaches you how to make your body beautiful and healthy with the least amount of effort. It then becomes a comfortable and efficient vehicle that allows you to be what you want to be. A controllable mind and sensitive, aware emotions are the practical benefits of Yoga. Yoga philosophy can help you get rid of boredom, frustration, useless anger, and intolerance, the negative emotional specters that haunt us in our lives. There is no need then to escape into the oblivion of alcohol or drug abuse, or to a fantasy leisureland where there is no contact with the real world. Drug abuse is not only a problem among the young. For example, the elderly use twice as much valium and seconal, the most widely prescribed tranquilizer and sedative, as the rest of Americans. Our elderly are sedating themselves right out of touch with reality.

"Too many older people are sedating themselves right out of touch with reality."

It is a well-known tenet of classical Yoga that we are our own best friend and our own worst enemy. You, as a Yoga student, learn to become friends with yourself, to stop doing the things that harm your mind and body and to recognize the limitations and benefits of age as simple facts, free from the emotional upsets which prevent their acceptance.

We as a nation must take action to change these destructive habits. When looking at life it is easy to be overwhelmed by all of the problems of mankind such as ill health, poverty, and fear. The total picture can seem so depressing that it is impossible for us as individuals to do anything about it. We need a starting point. The philosophy of Easy Does It Yoga gives the individual a foothold to reduce the seeming tragedy of existence to understandable human proportions. The practice of Yoga helps us to become stronger, more competent individuals, which enables us to find solutions to our own problems and thereby influence the entire community around us. This individuality is the essence of leadership in society, something we have been lacking in the United States recently, and which can come from older people.

Many would like to blame the government, society, their families, or big business for the condition of their lives. The philosophy of Easy Does It Yoga puts this responsibility squarely on the individual and says that you have two choices. One is to simply sit back, say that your life is over, and wait to die. The other is to do something meaningful to help yourself.

The choice is clear. We can either be rejected in old age as a passive, defeated, used-up cog in a giant wheel; or, by taking the responsibility to improve the quality of our own mental and physical health, we can become respected participants in the meaningful, intellectual life of our world.

5 WAYS TO INCREASE PERSONAL GROWTH

THROUGH THE PHILOSOPHY OF EASY DOES IT YOGA

As you get older it is essential that your mental horizons and awareness continue to grow and expand. In Easy Does It Yoga this is an integral aspect of total fitness. The Easy Does It Yoga philosophy, rather than outlining a specific dogma, creed, or rigid viewpoint of its own, challenges older people to explore perspectives of their own choice. The primary goal of Easy Does It Yoga philosophy is to awaken in older people everywhere a mature acceptance of the limitations of age as well as to develop an exciting and challenging mental attitude which fosters individual growth through the active pursuit of wisdom.

1. Live in the present.

Do not allow yourself to regress mentally into the past or worry about the future. Far too many older people reminisce about **what was** or fret about **what will be** instead of concentrating upon **what is.** Learn to live in the present. Decide how you can make today more constructive and satisfying by setting realistic daily goals and setting step-by-step work plans to achieve them. By doing this you will encourage self-growth and enjoy the happiness of feeling good about yourself each moment of every day.

2. Begin to study again.

Begin to study again. Form a study group among your friends that might replace one of those bridge games with an exciting intellectual challenge. Go back to school or enroll yourself in an adult education program. Explore new philosophies, comparative religions, mythologies, and psychological concepts, and organize group discussions to share your insights with friends.

3. Put ethical principles into practice.

Every week pick an ethical or moral principle, like truthfulness, compassion, generosity, freedom, or humility, or a concept expressed by a favorite religious or philosophical quote, and try to apply this idea in your everyday actions and relationships. By putting these ideas to the test in your actual living situation, you can begin to manifest in your personality the qualities which work for you.

4. Improve your mental health.

Mental health consists of harmonizing your actions with your thoughts and feelings. Your daily meditation will help you clarify your true desires and feelings. With this clarity it will be easier for you to keep your actions in harmony with how you actually want to behave.› behave.

5. Seek out challenging relationships.

Seek out young people and new relationships which will force you to examine new viewpoints and unfamiliar situations. As you meet these new experiences, try to step back from critical emotional reactions and refrain from making snap judgments which will inhibit communication. If you can open new lines of communication with people who have different ideas from your own, you will keep pace with the rapid changes in our society and allow younger people to benefit from your experience and wisdom.

SUGGESTED READING LIST

- **MYTHOLOGY**
  CAMPBELL. *Myths to Live By.* Bantam, 1972.
- **YOGA**
  CHRISTENSEN. *Light of Yoga.* The Light of Yoga Society, 1976.
  ELIADE. *Patanjali and Yoga.* Schocken, 1975.
  YOGANANDA. *Autobiography of a Yogi.* Self-Realization Fellowship, 1946.
- **PHILOSOPHY**
  CAPRA. *The Tao of Physics.* Bantam, 1975.
  DURANT. *Story of Philosophy.* Pocket, 1961.
  ZIMMER. *Philosophies of India.* Princeton, 1969.
- **WORLD RELIGIONS**
  GUILLAUME. *Islam.* Penguin, 1954.
  ISHERWOOD, ed. *The Bhagavad-Gita.* Vedanta, 1972.
  ISHERWOOD, ed. *The Sermon on the Mount According to Vedanta.* Vedanta, 1972.
  PONCE. *The Kabbalah.* Theosophical, 1978.
  PROGOFF, ed. *The Cloud of Unknowing.* Dell, 1973.
- **PSYCHOLOGY**
  COMFORT. *A Good Age.* Crown, 1976.
  FRANKL. *Man's Search for Meaning.* Beacon, 1963.
  GOULD. *Transformations.* Simon & Schuster, 1978.

"I'm thinking differently!"

"**I'm thinking differently.** I actually am. Is it possible that my thoughts could change? I think that I feel like I'm on a different plane or viewpoint of mind now. **I'm not as immature!** I was never able to communicate with younger people—I start to criticize or find fault or ridicule, and you know, one thing leads to another, and then they'd avoid me because they knew what my reactions always were. I was downright belligerent. Now it seems if I relax, my mental perception changes and **I'm not so critical. I'm smoother and calmer.** It surprises me—and them!"

Helen Gould
64
Euclid, Ohio

AUTHORS

●ALICE CHRISTENSEN. Alice is the founder and guiding force of The Light of Yoga Society and is one of the most remarkable women in America. She began her career in Yoga in the Spring of 1952 after an extraordinary series of what are now called paranormal, psychic, or spiritual experiences. Within a month her normal American life was abruptly and completely transformed by the force and light of Yoga which subsequently guided her to famous Yoga teachers like Swami Sivananda, Babaji, and finally to her Guru, Swami Rama.

An accomplished author and lecturer, Alice has written many books and articles on Yoga and is regarded as one of the foremost Yoga teachers in the world. Her sophisticated intellectual approach coupled with her professionalism and vast personal experience of Yoga are an inspiration to everyone who comes in contact with the LYS.

●DAVID RANKIN. David is both a Yogi of the highest caliber and an artist of equal acclaim. As one of the top watercolorists in the nation by the age of 18, David won a scholarship to the Cleveland Institute of Art. He began his Yoga practices with Alice and Swami Rama in 1967, and as Head of Teacher Training and Creative Director of the **LYS Video Arts Communications** Department, David's Yogic and artistic genius have since produced some of the most innovative teaching techniques, instructional manuals, videotapes, and Yoga publications in the field.

●THE LIGHT OF YOGA SOCIETY. Starting with a handful of interested and dedicated students, Alice began the LYS in the Summer of 1968. Since then the Society has expanded into a worldwide educational organization with Centers in the United States, France, and India. The LYS is rapidly setting the standard for excellence in Yoga instruction throughout the U.S. Its staff is constantly developing more effective ways to teach Yoga and creating teaching aids in all media which are recognized as the finest throughout the world.

● The entire staff of the LYS has been involved in the the production of the EDY manual and program. In particular, the following staff members have been indispensable: **Stephenson Grant** organizes and implements our research projects and designs our federal grant proposals; **Mary Robison** applies the EDY curriculum in the field and has contributed valuable additions and feedback to the program; and **Thomas Ball** assisted in the overall design and production of this book.

"The **Easy Does It Yoga** program has been a joy for us to design and implement, primarily because of the enthusiasm of our students. Seeing so many friendly faces light up with excitement as they explain to us what their Yoga has done for them has been an unforgettable experience for us. We wish you every success and encouragement as you begin to practice, and we want to help you in any way we can. If you have any questions or comments about **Easy Does It**, please write to us and let us know. **May the Light of Yoga Illumine your Life.**"

● Address correspondence to:
EASY DOES IT YOGA
The Light of Yoga Society
2134 Lee Road
Cleveland Heights, Ohio 44118

photo: Venice Gondolier